Lost Souls

Lost Souls

Women, Religion and Mental Illness in the Victorian Asylum

Diana Peschier

BLOOMSBURY ACADEMIC
LONDON • NEW YORK • OXFORD • NEW DELHI • SYDNEY

BLOOMSBURY ACADEMIC
Bloomsbury Publishing Plc
50 Bedford Square, London, WC1B 3DP, UK
1385 Broadway, New York, NY 10018, USA

BLOOMSBURY, BLOOMSBURY ACADEMIC and the Diana logo are trademarks
of Bloomsbury Publishing Plc

First published in Great Britain 2020

Cover design: Nick Evans
Cover image: Ellen Roche. Colney Hatch Asylum female case book, 1893–4,
London Metropolitan Archives.© London Metropolitan Archives

A catalogue record for this book is available from the British Library.

ISBN: HB: 978-1-7883-1807-5
ePDF: 978-1-7867-3660-4
eBook: 978-1-7867-2654-4

Series: International Library of Historical Studies

Typeset by Integra Software Services Pvt. Ltd.
Printed and bound in Great Britain

To find out more about our authors and books visit www.bloomsbury.com
and sign up for our newsletters.

For David and Francesca, with Love
And
For my Wonderful Fellow Volunteers at The
Listening Place, If Only This Charity Had Existed
in the Nineteenth Century.

Contents

Plates

Preface

I have oft seen the flower spring
From out the mould'ring wall –
I have seen the clusst'ring blossoms cling
And grace the ruined hall.

But here, 'mid scenes of human woe,
This little rose intends to blow.
So in life's shades, however drear,
Some ray of mercy will appear.

Bloom, tiny flower, a gracious hand
Invisible, unfolds thy leaves
O'er scenes of grief, by his command,
Joy still with sorrow interweaves.

Verses written by a woman confined as a lunatic in an asylum. They were addressed to a rose just budding into life, seen through the lattice window of her room. 1860.

> 'God will punish her: he might strike her dead in the midst of her tantrums, and then where would she go? … Say your prayers Miss Eyre, when you are by yourself; for if you don't repent, something bad might be permitted to come down the chimney, and fetch you away.'
>
> *Jane Eyre*, Chapter 2.

The words of Miss Abbot, Mrs Reed's lady's maid, strike a stern warning into the psyche of the young Jane Eyre following her imprisonment in 'The Red Room', a chamber where her uncle had died, as punishment for retaliating against her cousin John's cruelty and defying her aunt. Following a fit of passion, in which Jane describes herself as being 'out of herself', she says that 'Miss Abbot stood with folded arms, looking darkly and doubtfully on my face, as incredulous of my sanity.'[1] Jane is placed into a form of solitary confinement, locked in a room without heat or light, just like the 'seclusion' used in nineteenth-century mental asylums where the patient was removed from other inmates and placed in a darkened room, as light was seen as a source of irritation and darkness aided the calming of destructive or violent behaviour. Jane refers to having 'a consternation of soul' and says:

> How all my brain was in tumult, and all my heart in insurrection! Yet in what darkness, what ignorance, was the mental battle fought! I could not answer the ceaseless inward question – why I thus suffered …[2]

Jane's question about suffering was at the root of many females, Victorian mental asylum patients' belief that they must have transgressed the will of God. How else could they explain their feelings of psychological anguish?

The idea for this book originated in an episode of B.B.C. Radio 4's *All in the Mind*, a programme presented by the psychiatrist Raj Persaud. He mentioned that Bethlem Hospital had a wealth of patient records that would make an interesting study. Since then, researchers have made use of these case books[3] and some very scholarly work has been produced on the subject of Victorian asylums. This book is an examination of asylum inmates and their treatment, inspired by personal interest. More specifically, it is an exploration of how madwomen expressed themselves and how they were comprehended.

It soon became obvious that a comprehensive study of lunatic asylums in England would be impracticable and so I decided to limit my research to a selection of the larger county hospitals in and around London. Because the majority of patients in these asylums were Protestant, I have also looked at records of the Cork Asylum in Ireland, where most of the inmates would have been Roman Catholic, in order to discover any noticeable differences in the language used by the patients to describe their feelings.

This book examines case records of women in these nineteenth-century mental asylums and shows their gendered position within the institutions. The connection between physical and mental illness is explored through the theoretical texts of Victorian medical practitioners and actual diagnoses recorded in the asylum case books. Particular attention has been paid to the diagnostic categories of religious mania and religious excitement. Cases pertaining to the abuse of women, recorded, inferred and denounced in the press are examined and placed into context. Furthermore, this book aims to reveal the way in which madwomen employed the language of religion to express their perceived illnesses. In order to place these asylum records within a broader historical and social framework, the literature of the evangelical Sunday school movement has been examined. A sample of the asylum records for male patients has been scrutinized in order to demonstrate the differences between the feelings and language of male and female inmates and the divergence of treatment and understanding they received.

I have spent a lot of time with the case notes of 'mad' Victorian women, reading their stories and trying to make sense of them. Some of the records made me cry because they were so poignant. One entry that made a lasting impression was of a woman who was put into an asylum shortly after the birth of her baby, presumably suffering from postnatal depression. She died there many years later. All that was written about her after her initial admittance notes was: 'No visitors'. Other records described women who seemed to be more eccentric than mad and, if they had merely been accounts of out of the ordinary behaviour rather than the notes of females incarcerated in an asylum, they would have made me smile. One teenage girl was said to have refused her dinner because the parrot told her not to eat it, and an older woman caused disturbance to her landlady and neighbours by constantly accosting men and bringing them home for sex. This patient was convinced that she had an obstruction in her vagina and asked any man, who might be willing, to unblock it for her.

What I found in these narratives, as far as they went, was that the women were grappling with inexplicable feelings that they were struggling to put into words. In his book *Madness*, Roy Porter tells the story of some inspectors who were visiting an Irish lunatic asylum around 1850 when they were 'buttonholed' by an inmate alleging theft. What the man had actually said was: 'they took my language from me'.[4] In re-telling some of the women's stories in the light of nineteenth-century psychological thinking, attitudes towards women and above all, religious atmosphere, I hope to shed new light on these 'insane' working-class females.

The stories of middle- and upper-class women, who have been the subject of much nineteenth-century historical research, have largely been avoided. Statistics from annual reports and information about the day-to-day running of the asylums have been omitted as these too have been previously well

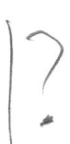

documented. The overall intention is to give a voice to the disenfranchised women who were put into the various asylums where they were frequently ignored and neglected and to establish that being female was a strong contributing factor to being diagnosed.

The vocabulary of madness is contentious and can cause upset and offence if used inappropriately. Victorian terms such as lunatic, madwoman, idiot and imbecile are unacceptable today and descriptions such as simple or weak-minded are no longer used. However, lunacy was the official word for madness in the nineteenth century and the above descriptors were used liberally in the asylum case notes I have looked at. Women were frequently seen as suffering from melancholy, various degrees of mania and hysteria. In the twenty-first century, the term 'mental illness' is more generally used for those suffering from psychological distress; however, this idiom suggests that 'madness' is an illness and this assumption is a problem for some people. Darian Leader, in recognizing the category of psychosis in psychology, made the following point:

> Recognising that there is such a thing as psychosis, however, does not mean that we need to buy into the discourse of mental health and illness. Although many people experience unbearable levels of suffering, this does not make them 'mentally ill', as there is simply no such thing as mental health.[5]

Barbara Taylor would agree with Leader when she stated:

> But is madness an illness? Most psychiatrists believe so, attributing it to glitches in brain chemistry. The fact that there is no compelling evidence for this has not prevented it from becoming a professional orthodoxy.[6]

The medicalization of madness began in the eighteenth century when it became envisaged as possible to treat by the medical establishment. By the nineteenth century it had become increasingly expanded upon by the men who specialized in this field were referred to as 'mind doctors', 'mad doctors' (a somewhat derogatory soubriquet) and more generally, 'alienists'. It was these doctors who applied a more humanitarian approach to the treatment of the insane, removed their chains and other constraints and, following the 1845 Lunatics Act, it was medicine that controlled the asylums rather than the keepers and owners of those establishments.

Throughout this book I have utilized the vocabulary describing madness as it appears in the asylum records and the writing of the 'experts' of the time. In a similar way, I have employed the language, particularly the religious idiom, used by the patients when they were attempting to communicate how they felt. I have used both nineteenth-century terminology around madness and the more palatable vocabulary of the twenty-first century because one of the aims of this book is to compare and contrast the value judgements of the Victorian era with some of those that still prevail in mental health services. The composition of the chapters is arranged around subject matter rather than being strictly chronological.

In order to put the research into asylum case notes into some kind of nineteenth-century context, they have been compared to the popular ideas of the madwoman found in imaginative literature of the time. The themes of loneliness, abandonment, heredity and other motifs were found in depictions of the Victorian madwoman as portrayed in some of the well-known and widely read novels of the day. The representations of madwomen in the work of such authors as Elizabeth Gaskell, Charlotte Brontë, Mary Elizabeth Braddon and Wilkie Collins were frequently wronged by society in general and men in particular. Novelists used their own experience and understanding of mental illness in their work so that it necessarily reflected contemporary ideas and medical opinion. Some characters and situations were based on 'real life' cases and writers like Rosina Bulwer Lytton actually recorded their own stories of ill use. By looking at actual case histories and comparing them with literary madwomen, this book will investigate whether discernible similarities can be observed between the real and the imagined.

As mentioned previously, the motivation behind the writing of this book is partially a personal response to a secret family tragedy. During the 1920s my own grandmother became mentally ill, she was diagnosed with 'acute mania' and, according to a woman who worked in my grandparent's house, she died screaming. Her death certificate indicates that she died from the after-effects of force feeding, a treatment that was administered in the privacy of her own home under the care of an aged, ex-prison physician. My grandmother's so-called treatment was in line with much of the medical care that was administered in the asylums during the nineteenth century, something I discovered during the course of my research for this book. Asylum records, specifically patients' case notes, which are less than a hundred years old, are closed to scholars for reasons of privacy and this limits the scope for comparison between centuries. Any references to incidents or situations from the twentieth and twenty-first centuries are taken from reports that are in the public domain or from personal experience.

Introduction: The Sin of Eve and Dangerous Emotions

One need not be a chamber to be haunted,
One need not be a house,
The brain has corridors surpassing,
Material place.

Far safer, of a midnight meeting
External ghost,
Than an interior confronting
That whiter host.

Emily Dickinson, *One Need Not Be a Chamber to Be Haunted* 1862.

It was, and to a certain extent, still is, a common perception that women are more susceptible to mental health problems than men. This 'feminization' of madness began to take hold in the Victorian era due to the re-defining of female nature and the representations of madness in art and literature that necessarily followed. Many nineteenth-century novelists dealt with madness in their books, as it was an important social issue of the day. Writers such as Charles Dickens, Charlotte and Emily Brontë, Anthony Trollope and Charles Reade used their personal experiences of mental illness in the depiction of their mentally unstable or insane characters. The construction of purpose-built asylums and the plethora of private madhouses that still existed at this time created an atmosphere of unease and a deep-seated fear of unlawful confinement. This was fuelled by sensational stories, both fictional and allegedly non-fictional. The nineteenth-century belief that madness was closely associated with femininity was demonstrated in scientific writing and popular discourse as well as in literature. Unmarried and middle-class women were believed to be more prone to mental disorders than women from the working-classes and in Victorian novels the madwoman became the vehicle for the manifestation of a suppressed life or frustrated sexual desire. It is extremely difficult to verify this perception from actual patient case notes as so many upper-and middle-class patients were placed in small, private asylums[1] and the records of these hospitals have largely been destroyed. However, following the implementation of the Lunatics Act 1845, for the first time all counties and principal boroughs of England and Wales were required to make provision for the care of lunatics. This led to an unprecedented period of mental hospital construction and an increase in facilities for the poor in the county asylums. The case books of these institutions contained evidence that showed that working-class women and those from an impoverished middle-class background were just as susceptible to mental illness as their financially better off sisters. This book will address four key areas that were vital to the understanding of the incarceration and treatment of women who were diagnosed as suffering from mental illness; namely, religion, education and moral and physical health.

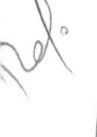

London and Co. Cork Asylums for the working classes

Bethlem Hospital records have proved to be a rich source of information as they are well preserved and more comprehensive than those of other London asylums. They were chosen for my study because of the clarity of the notes and because they mirrored the findings from other London asylums. Bethlem differed from the county asylums in that it had charitable status and was known to take middle-class patients who were easier to treat and more likely to recover. It was also a much older institution than any of the county asylums as it was the first, and for centuries the only, public institution for the care of the mentally disordered in England. The original Bethlem Hospital or 'Bedlam' was founded in 1247 as the Priory of St. Mary of Bethlehem. It has moved three times since its foundation. In 1676, Bethlem moved to a new building in Moorfields; this was the first custom-built hospital for the insane in the country. In the Victorian era it was situated at St. Georges Fields Southwark where the building still survives, now the Imperial War Museum.[2] In 1930, Bethlem moved to Monks Orchard in West Wickham where it still is today.

Hanwell Pauper and Lunatic Asylum, now known as St. Bernard's Hospital, was opened in 1831 as the First Middlesex County Asylum. It was a pioneering, purpose-built public asylum and still functions as an NHS psychiatric hospital. Its first superintendent, Dr William Charles Ellis (1780–1839), joined the hospital from his previous post running the West Riding Pauper Lunatic Asylum, while his wife, Mildred, became the matron. He had a reputation for advocating the humane treatment of lunatics, the application of moral therapy and his adherence to the principle of therapeutic employment. The asylum had its own carpentry, bakery and brewery and was, to a large extent, self-sufficient. Patients were encouraged to walk in the fresh air, and where possible, to work on the estate. The asylum very soon filled up and became overcrowded. The third superintendent of Hanwell, Dr John Conolly (1794–1860) made it the first large asylum to prohibit the use of mechanical restraints.

Colney Hatch Asylum, also known as the Middlesex County Pauper Lunatic Asylum, was opened in 1851 and was the largest asylum in Europe. Originally it followed the approach pioneered by Dr Conolly, which favoured the removal of restraints such as straightjackets and giving the patients work to do to alleviate boredom. It incorporated a large farm and workshops for tailoring and other trades. The asylum was built to house 1,000 inmates, but, like Hanwell, it soon became overcrowded. Extensions were added between 1857 and 1859 so that 2,000 patients could be housed; however, the staff could not cope with the influx of new patients and had to resort to the use of mechanical methods of restraint. Colney Hatch and Hanwell Asylum inmates were more working class than the majority of those in Bethlem and were less likely to be discharged 'cured'. Many patients remained in the hospital for a long time or until their death.

The Essex County Lunatic Asylum, the City of London Lunatic Asylum and Fair Mile Hospital were other hospitals which were established to treat the insane in and around London. The Essex County Lunatic Asylum, which later became Warley Hospital, was opened in 1853 in Brentwood, an area surrounded by fields and woods. The grounds were not laid out before the first patients arrived so that they might have some useful employment. The inmates were mainly drawn from the 'labouring poor' as the surrounding area was rural and poverty stricken. By 1860, the asylum was 'overfull'. Initially, mechanical restraint was employed for agitated patients, but its usage declined and, by the end of the nineteenth century, it was very rare. According to the records, most of the patients were considered incurable. Dr Henry Maudsley (1835–1918) spent a short time at the Essex Asylum as a medical officer when he was a young man. The City of London Lunatic Asylum, later Stone House Hospital, was originally constructed to provide for destitute, mentally ill patients from London. It opened in 1866 in Dartford, Kent, and included a working farm. In 1892 it took in private patients in order to improve its facilities. Fair Mile Hospital opened as the County Lunatic Asylum for Berkshire in 1870. It was a hospital for local people who were typically diagnosed as suffering from mania, melancholia and dementia. The patients, as in the other asylums referenced, were exposed to what was known as the 'moral regime'. Believed to be the best treatment for the insane, it included pleasant surroundings, fresh air, nourishing, plain food and occupation.

In 1845, a Westminster Act was enacted to create a District Asylum in Ireland, for the city and county of Cork. This new hospital replaced the old, inadequate one and was re-named Eglinton Asylum, after Lord Eglinton, the Lord Lieutenant of Ireland. It was opened in 1852 and the patients were mainly housewives, labouring classes, servants and unemployed. It was initially built to house 500 patients, and by 1900 the numbers had doubled. Ireland was a religious country and this influenced the admittances to the asylum. For example, unmarried mothers were sent there and made to 'wash away' their sins with tasks such as doing laundry for twelve hours a day.

Women's referrals and treatment

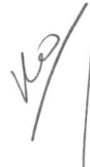

Asylum records from mainly the mid–late nineteenth century focused on what treatment the women received, what 'excited' their referral and what happened to them. This particular period was a new and more enlightened era for treatment of the insane which appears to have lasted for only a short time before the asylums became overcrowded and the 'horrors' of Victorian mental institutions, which have become legendary, ensued. However, the language employed by the women to express their feelings frequently led them being diagnosed as suffering from religious excitement or religious mania, as seen in Chapter 3.

The nineteenth century, according to scholars such as Elaine Showalter and Jane Ussher, saw what they term as 'the rise of the Victorian madwoman'. This occurred during the era when science and medicine were turning the old madhouses into hospitals for the insane and male psychologists were usurping the role of the asylum keepers who, in the past, had sometimes been women. As Showalter states, the medicalization of madness meant that:

> From the theoretical perspective, female psychiatric symptoms were interpreted according to a biological model of sex differences and associated with disorders of the uterus and the reproductive system. While physicians might pay attention to the contexts of the female complaint, such as poverty, the death of relative, or physical complications, they were totally indifferent to content.[3]

When women expressed unhappiness, fear, low self-esteem or anxiety, the doctors did not connect their emotions with what was actually going on in their lives. If they showed feelings of sexual desire, anger or aggression, these were perceived as not conforming to what was understood as proper feminine behaviour. The female life cycle, especially reproduction, was seen as dangerous for women's mental health, and therefore they were more vulnerable to insanity.

The psychological concept of hysteria was behind the diagnoses of many women seen to be suffering from some form of mental health problem. In the nineteenth century, emotion was seen as a force, 'adequate to the production of very serious disorders in the human frame, acting on the muscular, vascular, and secreting organs, and causing both of their structure and function.'[4] These 'disorders' were particularly female: 'these derangements are much more common in the female than in the male, … woman not only being more prone to emotions, but also more frequently under the necessity of endeavouring to conceal them.'[5] This concealment of emotion was specifically linked to sexual desire, as this was not seen as a fit or proper feeling for a woman. Such a theory appears to have led to some serious misjudgements in the treatment of women who were classed as hysterical when in fact they were physically ill. Robert Brudnell Carter (1828–1918), who was known for his theories and writing on hysteria, believed that hysterical girls were influenced by older women who had been examined with the speculum and treated with caustic soda for supposed uterine diseases. He maintained that these women loved to discuss their symptoms and narrated the sensations they experienced during examination and treatment which he believed they enjoyed, declaring, 'these patients would probably give the impression that a little leucorrhoea, a backache and a few blushing affirmatives to leading questions, would be deemed sufficient to justify an examination; and this might be expected to reveal abundant grounds for farther treatment'.[6]

Carter was outraged by the excessive use of the speculum, not because it was an invasive procedure against women, but because, as he put it, England was a nation where chastity and modesty were esteemed and practised. What he did not dispute was the idea that women could present with so-called uterine complaints, not because they were suffering from physical ailments, such as what has now been identified as endometriosis, but because they were seeking sexual gratification. This would seem perverse to a twenty-first-century reader, as would the Victorian use of Indian hemp or cannabis, in the treatment of gynaecological problems. 'The ladylike values of silence, decorum, taste, service, piety and gratitude, which Conolly[7] successfully imposed even on the wildest and most recalcitrant female maniacs, were made an integral part of the program of moral management of women in Victorian asylums. Within the asylums the experience of women would not be identical with that of men.'[8]

Practically pursuing these ideas around women's madness from the mid-nineteenth century, the use of surgery as a cure for mental disorders became quite common. Hysteria and other female disorders were frequently addressed by the use of hysterectomies and even clitoridectomies. The distinguished German psychiatrist Paul Flechsig (1847–1929) was known to have performed psycho-surgery on both sexes and his work in connection with women was outlined in his article on the gynaecological treatment of hysteria which was published in 1884.[9] Flechsig was professor of psychiatry at the University of Leipzig and head of the well-known psychiatric clinic at the same university. His reputation was worldwide. He was exposed by the German/American psychoanalyst William Niederland as having actually castrated women, by the removal of their reproductive organs, in order to cure what he diagnosed as their hysteria.[10]

The asylum should have been a place of refuge for women when they were at their most vulnerable. Popular literature fuelled the fear of false imprisonment and cruel treatment in the private mental hospitals that prospered during the nineteenth century and varied in size from a couple of patients boarding in a private dwelling house to the larger establishments such as Whitmore House in Hoxton, one of the Warburton family's London asylums. There were many scandals associated with private institutions, which purported to care for the mentally ill, and the latest and more enlightened thinking about mental health that became prevalent in the mid-nineteenth century saw the change from inmates of the asylums being seen as residents to being classed as patients. The new county lunatic asylums were to be regularly inspected on behalf of the Home Secretary and had a resident, qualified physician. The new regulations that came into force during the founding of the state-controlled county asylums should have ensured the safety of the inmates. Unfortunately, probably because of the defenceless position of women in madhouses, often without the support of friends and family, abuse continued to be a problem. Given society's attitude towards women, and madwomen in particular, it was hardly surprising that they were especially vulnerable to predatory men, be they keepers or fellow patients.

Women's susceptibility to mental illness

Charles Dickens wrote in *Household Words*[11] that: 'Female servants are, as it is well known, more frequently afflicted with lunacy than any other class of person.'[12] His explanation for this was that their social class and income made them more susceptible to mental illness than would be the case amongst the upper and middle classes. He also perceived governesses to be in danger of suffering from mental breakdown and, amongst other reasons which will be explored, their financial insecurity was seen as a major reason for their vulnerability. While the public asylums were over-subscribed by working-class women, most of the contemporary, nineteenth-century medical theory around Victorian women and insanity was focused on the middle and upper classes. It concentrated on feelings of suffocation by the patriarchal system and the intellectual and practical limitations of being a woman. However, there was a general acceptance by observers during that period that the poor were more likely to be diagnosed as insane than those on higher incomes. The reason for this class divide was most likely because there was a scarcity of material written by or about the hysterical female servant. Unlike her educated sisters such as Florence Nightingale or Charlotte Brontë, she would not have been given the opportunity to express herself to her doctors and lacked the education and time to record her feelings.

Part of the image of Victorian women showed them as being limited by their reproductive organs, restricted by their susceptibility to hysteria, sexual passion and fear and debilitated by the lack of a man in their life. Underlying all these masculine opinions on their mental and physical well-being was the biblical vision of Eve, the woman accused of being instrumental in the fall of man. This inherited sin of being female was an accepted belief amongst most Victorian women and coloured all their experience, especially when they were suffering. Even love was seen as a dangerous emotion for women because they were more sensitive than men, so, when a relationship went wrong it could, and did, cause serious mental damage. In 1838, William Willis Moseley, writing about the predisposing and exciting causes of insanity, said:

> Disappointed love has ruined the constitutions, broken down the mental powers, and inflicted more intense misery on a greater number of females, than LOVE ever made happy. The number which become nervous from this cause, is greater than from most others.[13]

This mode of thinking needs to be kept in mind during the assessment of women in mental hospitals at this time, in order to understand what was actually going on. To the post-feminist, twenty-first-century reader, many of the gendered assumptions will appear anomalous and outdated. However, in a society where being an 'old maid' could be seen as a predisposing condition to 'ovarian madness' or 'old maid's mania', a condition which made an elderly spinster believe that she was in love with an acquaintance of the opposite sex and that her feelings were reciprocated, they were considered perfectly normal. Disappointment in love, which often meant being jilted by the man she was going to marry, was frequently identified as the cause of a girl's mental breakdown as not only was she the victim of unrequited love but she was in danger of losing the precious status of being a married woman and a mother.

Religion and madness

Religion was used as a medium for control in the nineteenth century, particularly the control of middle- and working-class women. It was employed to instil fear into young girls by warning them of their fate should they choose to stray from the path allotted them by God. It is not surprising, therefore, to find that when a woman was suffering mentally, she often attributed her misery to some sin she had unknowingly committed.

How women and their mental and physical health were perceived by the 'mad doctors', the press, works of fiction and women themselves are all important in deciphering the female case notes of Victorian mental asylums. Another very significant aspect of these records was the way in which the women themselves interpreted their illness. The common language of females in these asylums was that of religion, with the emphasis on sin, lost souls and perdition. Sir George Henry Savage (1842–1921), the eminent Victorian psychiatrist, made a very interesting observation on the overemphasis on religion and how it coloured the language of people exhibiting symptoms of insanity. He noted that the religious and sexual sides of human nature were closely connected and that young, nervous females were particularly vulnerable to both of these very strong emotions. In a more measured and profound manner, he looked at theological hypotheses that formed much of nineteenth-century religious teaching and pointed out their close association with the feelings produced by a disturbed mind.

Savage indicated that a reason for the constant recurrence of religious ideas in the insane was that one of the most marked characteristics of religion was its mysticism; it professed to have dealings with powers which could not be weighed and measured. Religion had an enormous influence on the well-being of the individual; when a person passed from a condition of sanity into one of insanity, they experienced a series of indescribable feelings in which experiences might be rationalized as the powers of an omnipotent God. Savage clarified his theory by stating that religions had always sought to explain strange or unusual occurrences, and the same tendency was discerned in persons of unsound mind. In many cases, the patient suffering from the early stages of melancholy was searching for some possible cause of his/her misery. When they failed to find any satisfactory explanation in their bodily or mental surroundings, they turned to religion for enlightenment.[14]

John Conolly (1794–1866), another noted Victorian psychiatrist who introduced the principle of non-restraint of patients in mental asylums, stated in his 1854 lecture on the Character of Insanity that a trustful hope of a higher life after this life did not lead to mental derangement. In contradiction to this assertion, the study of nineteenth-century Sunday school literature that was produced for working-class girls observed that whilst the hope of a higher life might not lead to insanity, the fear of damnation and punishment for committing certain sins, imagined or otherwise, certainly added to the pain and confusion of both mental and physical illness.[15] Without specifically pinpointing what was considered unfeminine behaviour punishable by God, Conolly said that vehement passions, worldly ambition, frettings, envyings, jealousies and fits of wild, impulsive enthusiasm carried tumult to the brain and led to madness.[16] The case of Charlotte Wisdom (Bethlem 1822) illustrated this well.[17] Charlotte felt that if she were being punished by God for sins she had unwittingly committed, she might as well give herself up to all types of wickedness as her soul was already lost to the Devil. Foucault's assertion that Catholicism frequently provoked madness because it excited a fear of the 'Beyond' which was conjured up through the employment of fearful images and strong emotions which led men to despair and melancholia could also apply to the fear inculcated into young girls and women through religious instruction and church sermons.[18]

Education and madness

Education played an important part in determining the way in which young people understood the world around them and their designated place within that world. Given the popularity of the evangelical Sunday schools, the influence of the Sunday sermon and the rise of the non-Anglican, Protestant denominations, such teaching had an influence on the thoughts and feelings of young women with a very basic education. As religion interprets the spiritual, often inexplicable, world it is not surprising that its language was used by both men and women to explain their, otherwise mystifying, mental torment. Young, lower-class girls would have been familiar with their bibles and with religion in general.

By 1850, 2 million working-class children were enrolled in Sunday schools so their influence was fairly pervasive. The religious teaching of Sunday schools was thinly veiled social control designed to keep the young women, who toiled as maids and in other menial jobs, in their place. This schooling was gendered and added to the low opinion that so many troubled girls and women had of themselves, as noted by John Connolly. He saw that education was central to the formation and the strengthening of the mind, particularly important for women and young girls. He argued that insanity had its remote origin in imperfectly or misdirected education, especially referring to middle- and upper-class women who were not given the same level of education as their male equivalent. He was scathing in his opinion of the mind of the novel-reading female of whom he wrote:

> There is a frequent perversion of intellectual exercise, more fatal than its omission, which fills asylums with lady patients terrified by metaphysical translations, and bewildered by religious romances, and who have lost all custom of healthful exercise of body and mind.[19]

Religious education was injudicious in the way that it focused on sin and retribution. Many of the women in the county mental asylums may well have been scantily educated but, as Marit Fimland said of Charlotte Brontë, they would have had 'the Bible in their bones'.[20] Unfortunately, unlike Brontë, their ability to understand the use of religion as a method of social control would have been negligible or non-existent, and they were more inclined to take the words of the Bible literally.

Wives, Mothers and Abuse of Women in the Asylum

Women are more subject to melancholy impressions than men; their sedentary occupations, the powerful uterine sympathies that constantly act and react on their nervous system, their ready impressionability, added to the circumstance of their being essentially illogical, more naturally predisposes them to mental depression.

J.G. Millingen M.D., *Aphorisms on Insanity* 1840

In medicine, a woman's mental health was perceived to be closely connected to her bodily functions. As a result, they were admitted to asylums for dissimilar reasons from men and were consequently treated differently. Writing on the causes of insanity in 1868, Henry Maudsley stated:

> However it be that disorders of menstruation act, certain it is that they may exercise great influence on the causation and the cause of insanity. Most women are susceptible, irritable and capricious at that period … some exhibit a disturbance of character which almost amounts to disease; and, in the insane, exacerbations of the disease frequently occur at the menstrual periods. In a few rare cases, a sudden suppression of the menses has been followed by an outbreak of acute madness; but more frequently the suppression has occurred some time before the insanity, and acted as one link in the chain of causes.[1]

Maudsley also connected insanity with pregnancy, the menopause and uterine diseases, but his main concern was with 'the real internal disturbance produced in young girls at the time of puberty'.[2] Other doctors concurred with John Haslam (1785–1844), well known for his treatment of the insane, who wrote the following excerpt from his book on moral management of the insane, entitled *Feminine Confessions*:

> In females who become insane the disease is often connected with the peculiarities of their sex: of such circumstances those who are not of the medical profession would be unable to judge, and delicacy would prevent the relations from communicating with such persons. It ought to be fully understood that the education, character, and established habits of medical men, entitle them to the confidence of their patients: the most virtuous women unreservedly communicate to them their feelings and complaints, when they would shudder at imparting their disorders to a male of any other profession; or even to their own husbands. Medical science, associated with decorous manners, has generated this confidence, and rendered the practitioner the friend of the afflicted, and the depository of their secrets.[3]

By making women's insanity the result of some malfunction of their reproductive system, doctors such as Haslam put them into a unique category which was complicated by Victorian mores that prevented the open discussion of female bodily functions. In the above scenario, the doctor took on the role of the priest in hearing the woman's confession and in so doing either deliberately or inadvertently placed the female in the position of the sinner. As the depository of her secrets, the medical man assumed control over his patient and if he deemed her to be insane, he had the power to have her confined as a lunatic.

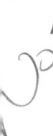

The moral management of lunatics, which concentrated on psychosocial care and lack of physical restraint, was applied differently to men and women. The close relationship between doctor and female patient, described by Haslam, changed their relationship from professional to personal. In calling specific consultations with women, 'Feminine Confessions', he associated the mind doctor with the Catholic priest and in the nineteenth century that was considered controversial.[4] The idea that women would talk intimately to a man about subjects that modesty prevented her from discussing with her husband or father, put the 'confessor' in a unique situation. It was suggested that the vocalization of such personal details could 'corrupt' a pure woman and put her under the control of a stranger, 'The confessors convey to the female mind the first foul breath which dims its virgin purity.'[5]

A further consideration in the treatment of female patients was that women were considered to have smaller brain capacity than men and were therefore deemed inferior to them. Skeletal sexual dimorphism was an important subject from the late eighteenth to the nineteenth centuries. Following the discrediting of the Galenic Theory of Humours, which had purported to show that females were disposed to lead a sedentary life, the Victorians needed a new, scientific validation of their ideas about women. They found this in early osteological studies, osteology being the study of skeletons and what they tell us about their lifestyle, sex, age and diet. Charles Darwin believed that men had larger brains than women and that this meant that 'man is more courageous, pugnacious and energetic than woman and has more inventive genius'.[6] He chose not to emphasize the fact that females have large brains relative to their body weight. Twentieth-century scholarship recognizes the misogynistic intent behind Darwin's ideas, 'the depiction of a smaller female skull was used to prove that women's intellectual capabilities were inferior to men's'.[7] This idea pervaded medical opinion as Alfred Beaumont Maddock writing in 1854 on the education of women observed:

> Without intending to enter into the oft-repeated argument of the relative superiority of the sexes, yet observation enables us to affirm, that in the higher powers of imagination, as well as in the severity and strictness of the reasoning faculties, the female mind must succumb to the larger scope and appliances of the male.[8]

Maddock's theories on the education and mental health of women he treated in his private asylum in Kent in the 1850s were clearly informed by his acceptance of the popular Victorian belief about diminished female brain capacity.[9] His book on mental and nervous disorders in the mid-nineteenth century shows there was a move towards improvement in the treatment and care of mental patients due to the 'new' theories on moral management. However, the sexual power dynamics between female patients and their male mind doctors were still important. This has been recognized by twentieth-century scholars:

> While there can be no question that women were better off in Victorian asylums than in the days before moral management, they were nonetheless subject to ubiquitous male authority. Furthermore, women's training to revere such authority in the family often made them devoted and grateful patients of fatherly asylum superintendents.[10]

Not only were women asylum inmates subservient to all men in authority but they worshipped a masculine God and a son of God with whom they had a very different relationship from that of their religious, male counterparts.[11]

In 1999, Leonard Smith wrote in his book *Cure Comfort and Safe Custody* that historians of the nineteenth century have tended to overlook the study of the patients who filled the institutions and have largely relied on generalizations or reproductions of statistics from annual reports.[12] In more recent studies, historians have examined actual case notes of Victorian mental asylums,[13] yet Smith's statement still retains a powerful element of accuracy. The neglect of patients' stories in the past may have been because many of the records were incomplete and tended to be just a few sentences after the initial admission notes. However, nineteenth-century medical opinions concerning mental illness were fairly well documented and it remains to identify how these ideas, particularly those regarding women, were being put into practice in the asylums.

Women, childbirth and insanity

According to the asylum records, during the mid–late Victorian era, mental illnesses that were specific to women became more defined. Women appeared to have been admitted at critical periods of their lives; they suffered from feelings of inadequacy, low esteem and subscribed to the belief in the inherent weakness of their sex. They expressed their deficiencies in terms of guilt and sin much more than the male patients did, although they found some solace in their relationship with God and particularly with Jesus. Under the umbrella term of 'mania', a term that was employed in the diagnosis of both male and female asylum patients, the more refined categories of hysteria and puerperal mania began to be common in pinpointing the reason for a woman's mental breakdown. Puerperal mania was believed, by alienists and obstetricians, to be a common cause of female insanity, which was usually manic. The condition was rarely mentioned by eighteenth-century practitioners and began to appear in medical texts in the 1820s and 1830s. Milton Hardy (1844–1905), medical superintendent of the Utah State Insane Asylum, defined puerperal insanity as developing 'during the time of and by the critical functions of gestation, parturition, or lactation, assuming maniacal or melancholic types in general'. He said that the condition presented 'a rapid sequence of psychic and somatic symptoms which are characteristic, not individually, but in their collective groupings'. These 'symptoms' included incessant, sometimes incoherent, talking, an abnormal state of excitement which meant that the patient could not sit or lie quietly, the inability to sleep and an aversion to the child or husband, which sometimes became homicidal. Patients were also observed to use obscene language and to behave in an indecent manner.[14] When women presented with these types of warning behaviours shortly after giving birth, they were acting in a manner that was at odds with the Victorian idea of female decorum and motherhood, something that would have contributed to their diagnosis.

Pregnancy and parturition were seen as being risky conditions that could affect women's psychological stability; this had a lot to do with the contemporary belief that for 'civilized' women, childbirth endangered both their physical and mental health. George Burrows (1801–1887), President of the Royal College of Surgeons and Physician to Queen Victoria, wrote that pregnancy and birth might prove detrimental to a woman's mental well-being and prefaced his theories with the assertion that women were more liable to insanity than men. The term 'puerperal insanity', which found its way into medical texts and language in the early nineteenth century, encompassed diverse forms of mental illness associated with childbirth and became a common nineteenth-century diagnosis.[15] Women's intrinsic biological weakness was seen to be paramount and George Savage (1842–1921), physician superintendent of Bethlem Hospital, noted that he believed that gender made a difference to the causation of insanity and he pointed to women's greater nervous instability as a reason for their susceptibility to madness in his work on *Insanity and Allied Neuroses* (1884):

> Women are more often upset by sexual troubles, and the periods of pregnancy, parturition, and lactation add gravely to the danger which they run of becoming insane. ... That there is an excess of female lunatics might be expected from the greater nervous instability of women, ... to the greater tendency of insanity to recur in women and the greater tendency of women to transmit insanity to their female children, who again are the more numerous.[16]

Women of childbearing age in the nineteenth century frequently had multiple pregnancies and were in danger of succumbing to puerperal fever due to the lack of knowledge about the transmission of bacteria and general hygiene. Puerperal insanity was a fairly common diagnosis at this time and a study by Sir John Batty Tuke (1835–1913), the eminent Scottish psychiatrist, *On the Statistics of Puerperal Insanity* (1865), found that over the period 1846–1864, 7.1 per cent of female admissions to the Edinburgh Royal Asylum were attributed to this condition. It was generally accepted that women had to use a great deal of mental as well as physical energy in the process of giving birth and so it followed that post-natal depression was a natural and biological side effect of pregnancy, labour and delivery. This condition was more generally known in the nineteenth century as post-partum depression or puerperal melancholia. Savage wrote that the symptoms of puerperal melancholia generally but not always came on later after delivery than attacks of puerperal mania: 'The onset of the disease being in every respect similar to the attacks of mania; sleeplessness, anxiety, and dread, being followed by delusions in reference to husband and children, and associated with hypochondriacal or other similar symptoms.'[17] Exhaustion from childbirth was given for the reason for Alice Mary Aphius's delusions when this 22-year-old married woman from Epping was admitted to Essex County Lunatic Asylum in March 1889. Alice declared herself to be in heaven even though she thought she had had committed some grievous sin. In her delusions, she thought that people gave her blood to drink and had turned her husband into a woman. Nonetheless, she was later discharged as 'improved'.

Sometimes, the female case notes mentioned 'puerperal causes' for a woman's attack of insanity almost as an incidental reason, ranking second or even third in importance behind such predisposing causes as religion or heredity. Yet, as previously noted, puerperal insanity was a recognized psychiatric diagnosis in the second half of the nineteenth century and alienists and obstetricians believed that childbirth was the common cause of a form of madness which was usually manic, serious and frequently fatal. Obviously, some of the patients labelled as suffering from puerperal mania were experiencing the delirium of fever caused by an infection. Often, though not always, the infection was the result of childbirth.

Some doctors attributed cases of mania to puerperal causes even when several years had passed since the patient had last given birth.[18] Forty-year-old Jemima Loune was admitted to Bethlem in May 1855, said to be suffering from 'religious enthusiasm' due to her religious delusions. She was a married, educated woman with four children, the youngest being eight years old. She had experienced her 'first attack' when she was thirty-two. Despite the diagnosis given on the certificate signed by her doctor, Samuel Griffith, Jemima's Bethlem case notes stated that her mental problem could be clearly traced to puerperal causes, as the first attack took place about six weeks after parturition. Why she should suddenly become delusional eight years later was not mentioned or even speculated on. It was almost as if a physical, 'female' reason was enough for her illness to be identified, allowing doctors a gendered diagnosis and for her to be treated accordingly. Although her notes state that her mother had died from a 'brain disease', this was apparently irrelevant to any diagnosis of Jemima. She was discharged four months later, declared 'cured'.

Another woman who was diagnosed as suffering from puerperal mania was 25-year-old Hephzibah Mary Williams, the wife of a joiner. There was no mention of her having suffered any other mental disturbance in the past, but nine days after the birth of her first child in January 1870 she was admitted to Bethlem, suicidal and delusional. Whilst pregnant, she had 'refused to eat for two weeks and had to be fed with a stomach pump', a brutal and often dangerous method of force feeding. She said that the child she was carrying was not hers and that she 'only had a lump of matter inside her'. Once she was delivered of her baby, she agreed that it was a child but that it had not come out of her.

Hephzibah's mental problems had started six months into her pregnancy. Her husband said that she had the 'startings up of religious melancholy' and she thought that she was damned. Hephzibah linked her early feelings of despondency to religion and thought she was being punished by God. Her mental health deteriorated until the point when she refused to eat, and tried to cut her own throat, jump out of the window and hurt those who tried to prevent her from committing suicide. She vowed 'to do for' the old nurse who attended her and was violent to her husband. Victorian psychiatrists recognized that pregnancy and lying in could precipitate mental illness as well as the actual act of giving birth, so the doctors at Bethlem identified Hephzibah's problem as being caused by her pregnancy and recorded it as a case of 'puerperal mania' with a strong suicidal impulse. It was noted that Hephzibah was in delicate health and refused coaxing to make her take her food. There was no mention as to whether the stomach pump was used in the asylum or indeed how Hephzibah was treated; however, she was given leave in June and was finally discharged, 'cured', in August, her recovery having taken seven months.

Death of children

Throughout their lives, Victorian working-class women dedicated themselves to their households and their families. They might have been almost continually pregnant from 'marriage' to menopause because of the virtual absence of contraception; however, the mortality rate of the infants who were born was high. Babies and children were at risk from dying from many diseases, such as smallpox, measles, whooping cough, diphtheria, dysentery and tuberculosis which alone, by the mid-nineteenth century, accounted for as many as 60,000 children's deaths every year. In 1864, the second main, moral reason for a female to be admitted to Colney Hatch Asylum was 'death of a child'.[19] Literature from the period reflected the prevalence of child deaths with the dead or dying child being a common motif in such novels as Charles Dickens's *The Old Curiosity Shop* (1841) and Thomas Hardy's *Tess of the D'Urbervilles* (1892).

Women in asylums had frequently been particularly affected by the loss of a child or children, but doctors often failed to recognize their sorrow as a primary cause of their depression. An example of this could be seen in the case of Ellen Smith who was a patient in Bethlem at the same time as Hephzibah Williams. Ellen was diagnosed with postnatal depression after she had tried to cut her throat with a razor, refused food and said that she believed she was wicked. Almost as an afterthought, her notes read that by the age of thirty-six Ellen had given birth to six children, all dead. Why her physicians did not deem it prudent to note down their consideration of the death of all her children in their diagnosis can only be guessed at, but it would seem that given the sheer amount of stillbirths during this period,[20] doctors gave little thought to its effect on the bereaved mother. Another example of how the death of a child could affect a mother can be seen in the case of Emma Mussell who was admitted to

Colney Hatch in 1856 because 'she sees ghosts who are constantly talking to her', refused food and was said to be 'harmless'. One month later, Emma's notes said that her husband had told them that fourteen years previously, when she was nineteen, Emma had had a child who was born dead. Presumably this was the beginning of the ongoing torment she was to suffer as a grief-stricken mother. A year after her admittance, Emma was discharged, 'cured'.

Unlike Ellen Smith, Eliza Miller's condition was recognized as being due to the death of her six-week-old baby when she became a patient at Colney Hatch in 1856. She was said to be 'of depressed spirits and of unsound mind'. She insisted that she had committed 'the unpardonable crime', but never confessed what this might be. It may have been her first attempt at suicide by dividing the vein in her arm, or maybe she felt guilty of the death of her child. As a result of her remorse, she attempted to hang herself; however, it is unclear if this attempt to kill herself was prior to her admission or the reason for it. Whilst still a patient in the asylum, in the dormitory where five other people were sleeping, Eliza killed herself during the night by slitting her own throat with a small, black handled knife with a five-inch long blade. A letter from her husband said that he could not find her birth certificate as she burned many papers before she was admitted. It was not mentioned why she, if it were she, felt the need to destroy the papers that documented her personal identity.

The continual bearing of many children took its toll on the Victorian wife as well as their constant care and the fear that they might fall ill and die. Ellen Penfold was a 28-year-old, Baptist dressmaker with five children, the youngest being under seven. She had lost five children in the last few years and talked about having 'committed great sins'. The fact that she was a Baptist facilitated her ability to convey her illness in religious terminology. She was self-destructive and claimed that 'she was dead and turned into dust'. She talked about heaven and subjects connected to religion, maintaining she had been to heaven, seen the Father and obtained pardon for her husband and children. Clearly Ellen was in distress possibly both mentally and physically; her use of religious language to express her suffering was effective and accessible to her carers.

Although the infant mortality rate was high in the Victorian era and the death of a child was more part of the 'natural order' than it is today, it was still seen as particularly tragic. Death in childhood was often romanticized in nineteenth-century society and it was not uncommon for parents to have post-mortem photographs taken of their children so that they had something to remember them by. Child death in fiction was also idealized as in Helen Burns in Charlotte Brontë's *Jane Eyre*, and Charles Dickens's deathbed scenes of Little Nell in *The Old Curiosity Shop*, Jo the crossing sweeper in *Bleak House* and Paul Dombey in *Dombey and Son*. Whatever the novelists and evangelical story writers wrote, it reflected the grief experienced by the parents, particularly the mother, over the loss of their child. However, although puerperal hysteria was usually identified, the impact of the death of a child or children was frequently overlooked by asylum doctors.

Depression following a stillbirth or several stillbirths, which was, as previously noted, a common occurrence in the nineteenth century, could, and often did, lead to suicidal thoughts and attempts. This was a specifically female complaint and restoring the woman to her marital and housewifely duties was seen as of paramount importance. In June 1873, twenty-three-year-old Mary Tomlin, the wife of a labourer, was taken into the Fair Mile Mental Hospital having been in a 'state of insanity' for about six months, registered as both suicidal and dangerous. The cause of her madness was unknown, but as it was recorded that some of her family had been insane, Mary's problems appeared to have been attributed more to heredity than to the fact that she had had three stillborn children. The last one had been born just a few months previously, just before the onset of her breakdown. Mary was said to be 'labouring under religious delusions' having said that she saw 'Jesus Christ distributing loaves and fishes in Buckland Church on Sunday last', that she was 'possessed by a devil' and 'he would never let her have a live child again'. Mary's mother-in-law appeared to be far from sympathetic to this poor young woman's despair at having produced three dead babies, stating that her daughter-in-law was 'at times incoherent', that she would 'not perform her household duties' and she 'threatened her husband's life continually'. The only further knowledge we have of Mary Tomlin was that she was 'exceedingly robust and stout and her whole body was loaded with fat'. Whether she was eventually discharged into the care of her family is unknown.

Anxiety around children whether it be their death, illness, fear for their well-being or even guilt at having procured an abortion was seen again and again in the female case notes of women in Victorian asylums. These motherly concerns were necessarily gendered given the physical demands of childbirth on a woman's body and the concerns of women for their offspring. Sometimes the male doctors recognized what was behind the cause of the woman's suffering, but not always. It remained a matter of speculation, however, whether this was by choice or ignorance. One case, from the early half of the century, demonstrated an understanding and kindly attitude towards a mother's angst even though it might seem patronizing in the twenty-first century. Dorothy Margerum was forty years old and single. She had one child living, but she imagined that her child was starving to death. Everything she ate she felt her child ought to have and she therefore 'took her provisions with the greatest reluctance'. It frequently became necessary to 'administer, by force, the sustenance which she obstinately refused to take of her own accord'. This reluctance to eat had reduced her to almost a skeleton. Reading between the lines of this report, it was logical to surmise that Dorothy had had other children die, probably from malnutrition, and evidence that coping as a single mother in early Victorian England was very hard. A comment from her doctor read: 'the poor creature suffers in her mind all the anguish of maternal woe.' It was also noted that she was quite harmless and at no time 'inclined to be mischievous'. Regrettably nothing more was written concerning Dorothy, her child, or if she survived the force feeding.

The loss or fear for the safety of children could, as we have seen, cause a woman great distress even to the point of taking her own life. The case of Martha Ann Slater was one of a childless woman who nevertheless suffered severe mental disturbance because she believed that she had been the cause of a child's death. When she was in her late thirties, she had been admitted to the asylum following her first 'attack' of insanity. It is possible that she had lost her own child and this had been the onset of her delusions. By the time she was sixty, Martha had been working as a servant when she was again admitted to Bethlem in 1858. She imagined herself to be 'lost' and continually 'prompted by evil spirits to do some dreadful acts'. To prevent this happening she felt that she must frequently fall to her knees. She was very melancholy and had a great fear of dying in consequence of her sinfulness as she believed she had killed a child who was entrusted to her care. As Martha was both a servant and childless she would probably have been a useful child minder. Working women without older children or other relatives to provide childcare might pay a neighbour or other available woman or girl to do the job. In middle-class Victorian families, servants assisted with the rearing of children and were often liable for their nurture. However, for Martha, the belief that she was culpable for the death of a child was unfounded as the child in question had actually died of measles in its mother's house. What caused Martha to have such a disturbing fantasy concerning the death of a child was not explored and she died in the asylum, uncured, a year later.

It was not the prerogative of any class to suffer more than the other where children were concerned, but maybe the middle and upper classes were better understood by their doctors, because they were believed to have more sensitive natures than working-class women. Private asylums, such as Ticehurst House Hospital in Sussex which accommodated the gentry, were more likely to have included middle-class patients. Mary Ann Burnett, a gentlewoman and wife of a publisher, was admitted to Ticehurst in 1865 following a suicide attempt. It was recorded that she had previously attempted to bleed herself to death by 'puncturing the veins in the back of either arm with a penknife' and the wounds were still open and visible. She had also attempted to poison herself with laudanum and to throw herself out of the window. She concealed a razor in her pocket with the intention of 'destroying herself', but was detected and prevented. Mary Ann was said to be quite 'incoherent in her conversation'. Finally, after attending service with her husband, whilst he was engaged talking to an acquaintance, Mary Ann 'ran off down a dark alley and made a most determined attempt to cut her throat'. She inflicted several wounds on herself, 'dividing the trachea at its junction with the larynx'; she cut from ear to ear. It was clear that Mary Ann was determined to commit suicide. It became apparent that she was so overcome by grief because she had recently lost her only two children; the last, a most accomplished girl aged fifteen, had died just three months previously. Since then, she dwelled on the death of her children and insisted that she wished to join them. Having failed to kill herself, Mary Ann believed that she had been too wicked for God to forgive her.

Suicide was taboo in Victorian times and severely condemned by religion. Christianity viewed it as a serious sin because it broke the sixth commandment, 'thou shall not kill', and allowed no time for repentance. One of the most important tenets of Christian belief, the sanctity of human life, was violated by suicide, and 'self-murder' was a mortal sin in the eyes of the church. Suicide or the crime of 'felo de se' was, strictly speaking, against the law, although there was much debate around the medicalization of the act. In the case of Mary Ann Burnett above, she believed that justice would pursue her and that she would have to be removed to prison for attempting her own life. She had become the victim of her belief in God and the afterlife. In wishing to join her children in heaven, where she clearly believed them to be, she had broken the law of God that prohibited self-killing and the law of the land that was based on Christian doctrine. In being admitted to a mental asylum she had, at least, avoided the punishment of imprisonment and the shame of a trial.

The anguish of mothers and wives

Shame, guilt and worry made mothers mentally ill and often suicidal. They were inclined to feel that it must be their fault if their child suffered and they were being punished by God. These overpowering feelings of despair could be observed in 23-year-old Jane Emma Hill, a moderately educated milliner who was admitted to Bethlem in 1861, having become suicidal and depressed due to the shame of having an illegitimate child. She was found to be in 'poor bodily health', which suggested that she was finding it difficult to cope with her child. She would 'sit perfectly still, her eyes fixed upon the ground' and would not reply to any questions put to her. Her aspect was 'extremely melancholic', 'she appeared to neglect her person', and would only take food when force was used. She had made five or six attempts to take her life, by using a knife and by attempting to stab herself in the throat with a pair of scissors. Her recuperation was lengthy, but she gradually improved and after a year she was fit enough to be discharged. What happened to her child was not documented. The Victorians placed great importance on marriage, and those who deviated from this social norm faced condemnation by their families and communities. The mother of an illegitimate child was made to feel such shame that it was not uncommon for her to abandon her infant or give it up to 'baby farmers' who specialized in the systematic murder of illegitimate babies.[21]

Like suicide, the taking of an unborn life was also taboo at this time; however, there is no doubt that some women aborted their unwanted babies. In an era where there was no reliable form of contraception, sexual intercourse frequently resulted in pregnancy. If the single mother was also the sole breadwinner, the presence of an illegitimate child could lead to her losing her job, resulting in starvation and even death. The religious and cultural memes of chastity and purity were used by society as powerful deterrents. Charles Dickens summed up the fate of the orphaned, illegitimate child in his novel *Oliver Twist*: 'A parish child – the orphan of a workhouse – the humble, half-starved drudge – to be cuffed and buffeted through the world – despised by all, and pitied by none'.[22] The stigma of illegitimacy applied to both the unmarried mother and her offspring and this situation was exacerbated by the 1834 Poor Law containing the Bastardy Clause which was drawn up to be very much in keeping with nineteenth-century evangelical Christian teaching. It absolved the putative father of responsibility for his child and socially and economically victimized the mother in an effort to restore female morality. In other words, the new law singled out women alone to face the humiliation of having a child out of wedlock.[23] The notion of heredity played an important part in the treatment of illegitimate children, in a similar way to how it was perceived as an important factor in the diagnosis of madness. Children conceived outside the bonds of marriage were deemed to have inherited their parents' lack of moral character. Thus, the majority of orphanages refused the admittance of illegitimate orphans as they feared they might contaminate the minds and morals of the legitimate children. Even in the workhouse, single mothers were kept apart from women and girls of 'good character'.

It was not only single women who were distressed at finding themselves pregnant. Some married, working-class women did not welcome the idea of another mouth to feed and it was common for them to procure an abortion for an unwanted pregnancy; it was a useful form of contraception. Abortion had been illegal and punishable by law in England since 1803 and The Offences against the Persons Act (1861) created the new crime of obtaining the means of carrying out a termination. These were usually poison and specific instruments. Because of its legal status, abortion was driven underground and there were many 'back-street' abortionists. The Christian Church condemned abortion and the women who underwent the procedure were going against the moral teaching they had received. This meant that they were frequently left disturbed by feelings of sin and guilt for what they had done. Sometimes these negative emotions were strong enough to cause a woman to experience a mental breakdown.

This would seem to have been the problem with 36-year-old Charlotte Kelsey, a painter's wife, with two children, the youngest being three. She was recorded as having had an 'attack' when she was sixteen which had been caused by a sudden fright. When she was admitted to Bethlem in 1855, she was diagnosed as suffering from 'religious excitement'. Charlotte believed that she was 'doomed to hell', could already feel the 'onset of her agonies' and that 'the devil frequently leapt upon her'. She 'fancied' that she had 'offended' God by 'taking some medicine several months previously' and had lost all hope of eternal salvation. It is possible that Charlotte had taken some concoction to bring on an abortion. As a working-class woman who already had two children, this would not have been unlikely nor would the suffering caused by the loss of her baby and her conscience later on. Seemingly, Charlotte could not come to terms with what she had done and it was recorded that several months after her admittance, she was given four weeks' leave to return home, and she was then discharged 'uncured'.

Women who conformed to the Victorian ideal of marriage and motherhood could not always escape violence from their husbands. This could be another cause of mental breakdown and admittance to a lunatic asylum. Poor women faced tremendous challenges in keeping their households together, and they were expected to accept the self-sacrifices that this required, even when it meant suffering physical abuse.

Maria Brindley, the 29-year-old wife of a cabman, had been insane for two years and the cause of her insanity had been put down to 'ill treatment by her husband'. There was even physical proof of this as she had a black eye the day she entered Colney Hatch in 1853 suffering from 'mania'. Maria had found her husband in bed with her sister, and since then her jealousy and his abuse were thought to be responsible for her strong suicidal tendency. As if the betrayal by her husband and her sister were not seemingly enough to cause her illness, Maria's notes tell us that her father was insane. Parental insanity seems to occur in patent's records, often as proof of their susceptibility to madness, in addition to the overriding instigating causes for their insanity. It appears that she had remained with an abusive husband because of the children but it had all proved too much for her and she had ended up in a mental asylum.

Emma Kemp was also recorded as suffering from mania when she was in Bethlem in 1856, and because she believed herself to be the 'vilest sinner' hers was deemed to be 'religious mania'. In reality, she had been abused by her husband who, according to Emma's sister, treated her cruelly and beat her. This young woman had a child aged five months and was in such a bad state that she had been put under restraint before entering the asylum. Whilst there, she was confined to bed by way of detainment for several weeks. Her fear for herself and her little child may have been enough to make her retreat into the protection of her religion, surfacing in her mania. Women have a history of taking on the blame for the abuse of others and this would account for her seeing herself as a 'vile sinner'.[24] Emma was kept in Bethlem for six months and there is no record as to who had charge of her baby; she was then discharged, 'cured'. Her case notes do not reveal where she went, but the chances were that she had to return to her husband.

In Victorian England, women were second-class citizens and this was particularly true for married women. On marriage, a girl would pass from the authority of her father to that of her husband. Under the law, a woman was subjugated to her husband, and he had control over her earnings, her property, her children and even over her own person. These rights meant that a husband could beat his wife almost with impunity, only if he went too far or if his wife resorted to the police because of serious injury, could a man be taken to task. Women, working-class women in particular, saw it as their lot in life to be the recipients of men's violence and should they complain, they were not viewed with any sympathy by members of their community. Because a man had the right to 'chastise' his wife, it was difficult for the woman to prove that his punishment of her had not been justified. A woman was also, understandably, afraid of making a complaint against her husband as he might attempt to take his revenge on her. Amongst the poorer members of society, domestic cruelty could be triggered by bad housing conditions, drink and unemployment.

Unrequited love and women's mental health

Women were also seen as being more susceptible to mental health problems because of their capacity to fall in love. As J.G. Millingen observed in *Aphorisms on Insanity*: 'Religion and love, two sentiments closely akin are the principal sources of their (women's) melancholic monomania'. He was not alone in seeing love, in particular unrequited love, as a peculiarly female malady. This condition was usually referred to as 'disappointment in love' in the asylum case books and was the instigating cause of much mental illness. William Willis Moseley's treatise on *Predisposing and Exciting Causes of Insanity* (1838) spelt out the dangers: 'Disappointed love has ruined the constitutions, broken down the mental power, and inflicted more intense misery on a greater number of females than love ever made happy. The number which became nervous from this cause, is greater than most others.'[25] In nineteenth-century literature, possibly the most famous example of disappointment is Miss Havisham in Charles Dickens's *Great Expectations*. The mental breakdown she suffers after she is jilted by her fiancé develops into a madness that ruins her life and poisons the lives of those around her. The cases of disappointment found in the County Asylums during this period were rather more prosaic than that of a woman in her wedding dress living in a decaying mansion where the ruins of her wedding breakfast still sat mouldering on the table. They were, nevertheless, in their own way, poignant and the assumption that the demise of a love affair, real or imagined, could cause insanity was invariably gendered. This premise was reinforced by George Savage, the eminent and fashionable consultant on mental diseases, who said: 'The persons most likely to break down from disappointed affections are women; and the danger increases with age up to a certain limit, so that it would be considered a much more serious thing for a woman of thirty to be cast off by her lover than for one of twenty.'[26]

Disappointment in love or the hope of marriage was frequently seen as a main or contributory cause of mental breakdown in women and it was commonly linked with religious mania. In a society that held that marriage and childbearing were the ultimate goals of every female and made a woman's life meaningful, it was obviously difficult when that future was taken away from her. Unrequited love inevitably had a serious detrimental effect on some women's mental health and whilst this may have been true of men as well, Victorian psychiatry and society had a different opinion on how, and by what means, men's mental health was affected; 'disappointment in love' would not have been seen as a masculine emotion, especially for working-class men. An early example of 'imagined' love can be found in the case of Susan Morgan who was admitted to Bethlem in 1821 as a victim of 'religious superstition'. Susan was twenty-nine and a cook in a respectable family when she received, what she referred to as, her 'call'. From that moment on she 'lapsed into distraction and wild enthusiasm'. Susan believed that she was with child by a man with whom she had been many times. His name was omitted for her case notes and replaced with a blank space, indicating that it had been 'censored'. In the asylum she was clean, 'regular', usually a reference to moderate, controlled behaviour, and inoffensive, so she was discharged, 'well', ten months later. Tragically, back home she became deranged again and drowned herself in a fit of despondency. In Susan's case notes there was no suggestion that she might have been telling the truth about the man she had named as her lover. He was kept anonymous which might have suggested that he was of a higher rank than her. It is not clear whether Susan was really pregnant or imagined. Whatever the truth of her situation, she could not cope with the rejection and felt that her only solution was to commit suicide.

Rejection in love had also affected another woman, forty-year-old Ann May, a single dressmaker. Ann's brother explained her mental condition by recounting her history. She was 'seduced at eighteen years of age by a gentleman of rank' with whom she lived in a 'state of concubinage' for twenty years, then the gentleman married and 'terminated all connection with her'. Ann became distraught and suffered 'great distress in her mind' and, having nowhere to live, returned to her childhood neighbourhood where she still had relatives and ultimately joined the Wesleyan Society. She was very 'zealous in her attendance upon various classes, prayer meetings and chapel services', so much so that she was admired by a church leader who paid her a lot of attention and was regarded by herself and her family as her future husband. This courtship proceeded for some time, until, possibly because her previous love affair became known to the church leader, he 'discontinued his attentions'. Ann did not demonstrate undue distress at this time. In fact, she appeared more cheerful than usual towards her relatives; however, they noticed that she was 'unusually garrulous and passed whole nights in sewing and other occupations of millinery'. Her conduct became so eccentric that it seriously worried her friends and they feared she was not right in her mind. She became quarrelsome and violent, tore her clothes and destroyed furniture and was eventually removed to the workhouse at Chelsea and from there, in 1850, to the Hanwell Asylum. She was said to be an imbecile, suffering from general paralysis. She was prone to such violence that she had to be restrained; however, she was very strong and managed to fracture her leg whilst kicking out. When the attendants bound up her broken limb and tried to stabilize it, she repeatedly tore off the bandages and splint.

Ann was diagnosed as having general paralysis, a condition caused by late-stage syphilis and her symptoms described would have certainly confirmed that opinion. General paralysis of the insane was the outcome of untreated syphilis. It was identified as a disease in the early 1800s, but its link with syphilis was not fully established until the turn of the century. It was a diagnosis more commonly found in male asylum inmates, typically in their thirties or forties, and was frequently manifested in grandiose delusions and unruly behaviour. When the disease was detected in women, they were said to be prostitutes or innocent victims infected by their promiscuous husbands. It was associated with working-class women rather than the genteel, middle and upper classes.[27] In the case of Ann May, having been taken as the mistress of a 'gentleman of rank' when she was only eighteen, it must be assumed that it was he who had infected her. Historically, syphilis was very difficult to cure. Before the development of penicillin in the 1940s, mercury was frequently used in its treatment. However, because Victorians associated syphilis with prostitution, the disease carried a social stigma. As a result, women who displayed signs of the infection were often not informed by the doctor what their symptoms signified as this would necessarily imply that they had been infected by their husband or lover. Physicians were wary of breaking the confidentiality of a man, who was usually the person who paid their bills, even if they suspected him of immoral conduct. If the ulcers caused by syphilis were not treated, the bacteria could move through the body and in the late stages often affected the brain and caused mental disorders. Nineteenth-century doctors held the theory that syphilis was hereditary. A woman with the disease could pass it to the next generation, which made it a threat to society and disgraced the female carrier even more. Ann's failed love affair with the church leader only exacerbated her distress, both mental and physical. She must be seen as the exploited victim of a debauched man who cast her off when she was no longer of any interest to him. She was fortunate that her family took her in and tried to help her make a new life, but sadly it was too late.

Colney Hatch asylum had many young working-class girls admitted in the mid-nineteenth century because they had broken down mentally due to rejection or abandonment in love or marriage. This went against the, previously mentioned, perception that melancholy, brought about by failure in love, was mainly a middle-class female complaint. Just a few cases found in the Victorian case books include, Jane Blyne Hilliard, a parlour maid; Elizabeth Coventry, a domestic servant who spent eight years in the hospital and subsequently died; Esther Kitchingman, a fishing tackle maker; Frances Mercy Adenham, who spent nineteen years incarcerated before being discharged; and Sarah Ann Yonwin, who was in good health when she was admitted, but died a year later on Christmas day. Sometimes the 'insane' girl had been abandoned by the lover she had been living with, as Martha Lloyd, a matchbox maker from Bethnal Green. She, like Sarah Ann Yonwin, was said to be in good physical health when she entered Colney Hatch, but she died two years later. Charlotte Webb, a chenille net maker, who suffered from melancholia following a failed love affair, also died soon after admittance.

Love, in many different guises, was seen as particularly troublesome for women's mental health, whether it was unrequited, abusive or unwanted attention. It could even, as in the case of Rhoda Chandler, have been 'over excitement'. Rhoda was a stout, healthy-looking daughter of a baker from Edenbridge in Kent. She was admitted to Bethlem in June 1855 because she was delusional, suicidal and was considered a danger to others. The reason for her mental unrest, which was supported by her case notes, was given as 'excitement at a proposal of marriage from a man she had long had an affection for'. Why this longed-for proposal should have made Rhoda temporarily insane was not explained, all that was recorded was that she was discharged in March 1856, 'cured'. We can only hope that her fiancé was willing to wait for eight months whilst she got over her excitement and that they lived a long and happy married life.

The unfeminine Victorian eccentric

During the nineteenth century, the lines between madness and eccentricity were often blurred. However, when a woman stepped outside the social conventions of the day or failed to fit into the Victorian ideal of femininity, they could find themselves in a mental asylum. This happened to Elizabeth James, a woman who was far from modest, dainty and submissive and may have suffered the loss of a child or been deserted by her husband.

Described as being a lady of great personal magnitude, Elizabeth James[28] lived for fourteen years in Canterbury Place in Lambeth where she was as well known for her eccentricities as for the state of her dilapidated mansion and the 'clamorous attention paid to her by arch boys and idle gazers'. Various reports circulated as to the cause of her insanity; some stated that she was deserted by her husband and others that her child died by getting into a copper of boiling water due to the carelessness of his nurse. Whatever the reason, Elizabeth's eccentricities became a complete nuisance to the other residents in her neighbourhood who particularly took exception to the state of her house. Her strange behaviour took many different forms; the neglected maintenance of her home resulted in every window in the front being left unrepaired and the railings missing. She lived alone without a servant or a companion though she had a charwoman to clean the part of the house that she lived in. She cooked her own provisions, enjoyed the best of everything, so was obviously not without means, and what she could not eat she threw into the fire. She was accustomed to 'parade in front of her house as a sentinel with her head adorned with a turban *à la Turque* and a quarterstaff in her hand'.

Elizabeth was given a room in the criminal wing of the asylum which was well furnished with her own things and she was allowed to buy what food she wanted. She was addicted to 'strong liquor' which was given as one of the reasons for her disorderly conduct. However, she was not allowed to drink alcohol in Bethlem and her disorder continued. She styled herself as a woman of great scientific knowledge, but also had religious delusions and believed that she was the daughter of the Almighty. When she was displeased she would look upward and exclaim: 'Joe! Joe! Do you think this is right? Is this justice? Is this justice Joe?' Not much more was known about this extraordinary character except that sometimes she was inclined to violence but had done no particular harm. She was a well-educated woman who owned some property and was said to have been 'honest in her dealings' and 'punctual in her payments'. Despite her odd ways, she obviously had some coherent financial sense as she used to 'attend the bank to receive her dividends with great punctuality and paid her bills correctly'.

One aspect of Elizabeth that would have made her more noticeable than other women was her manly appearance; she was a huge size with masculine features and had more the 'voice of a stentor' than an 'accomplished fair one'. Mobs frequently gathered and this annoyed her and her neighbours, so she would sometimes 'sally forth and distribute her sturdy forearms indiscriminately upon the heads and shoulders of the gazers'. When she went out for a walk, she carried a brass ladle concealed in her muff and she was always joined by the 'arch boys', or as she called them – her 'jolly crew' – but if annoyed or attacked by them she would draw her ladle and 'baste them soundly'. Elizabeth would go around town in all sorts of strange outfits, leopard skin apron, odd looking furs, tippets, muffs, shawls and cloaks. She was always followed, even though she did not like to be. 'One of her Amazonian freaks procured her an assignment to Horsemonger Lane Prison for riotous conduct'. From there she was sent to Bethlem. The physical description of Elizabeth James along with her unfeminine comportment would have been a factor in her being diagnosed as insane. Women were supposed to conduct themselves along the lines of prescribed Victorian femininity and to do otherwise was seen as aberrant.

Another patient in Bethlem in 1822, who did not fit the Victorian ideal of femininity, was Charlotte Dully, a 45-year-old, married woman who 'fancied herself to be a man'. 'She sometimes styled herself as a boy. When spoken to she bowed and scraped and put her hand to her head in every respect like a footman'. Charlotte was said to be particularly attached to the matron whom she called 'my beauty' and was quite uneasy every day until she saw her. Apart from her masculine tendencies, Charlotte's notes said that there was nothing else remarkable in her manner. She was orderly, clean in her person and habits, perfectly quiet and harmless. Charlotte obviously failed to conform to Victorian society's expectations of female conduct to the extent that she was deemed mentally disturbed and considered abnormal.

The diagnosis and treatment of madness has always been gendered but it depended on the century in which the 'madwoman' lived as to how that insanity was dealt with. Some aspects of what is perceived as women's madness are constantly reinterpreted according to the social mores of the era. As the modern day psychologist and historian Jane Ussher has so succinctly put it:

> When I was an adolescent my mother was mad. Because it was the 1970s, she was deemed to be afflicted by her 'nerves'. Had it been 100 years ago, she would probably have been called 'hysterical' or 'neurasthenic'. Today, it might be 'post-natal depression'. … her unhappiness, pain and fear resulted in withdrawal, apathy, tiredness and a sense of worthlessness.[29]

When she tried to commit suicide, Ussher's mother was deemed mad enough to be taken to the local mental hospital. Having tried to contain her anger and frustration, she had turned it in on herself. This 'turning in on oneself' is a particularly feminine trait as is taking the blame for one's mental health problems. In the nineteenth century, women's behaviour and the way they reacted to their circumstances were closely prescribed. To stray from what was considered to be the feminine standard could indicate madness, as could the physical complications and limitations of being a woman. Because of this, the fear of insanity was always something that threatened women and could be, and was, used as a contrivance to control them. In particular, love was considered a dangerous emotion for a female and when it was misplaced, it could be as damaging as when it was unrequited or abused. Madness was not simply a diagnosis for women; it was an instrument of manipulation and management to force them back into their allotted roles.

Sexual abuse in the asylum

Once a woman was admitted to a mental hospital, even a county asylum, she was not necessarily protected and incidents of sexual abuse could be detected in the female patients' records. Sometimes they were overt, whilst others were more 'implied'; for example, in the collection of photos from the Hanwell Asylum, one patient was pictured holding a very young baby but there was no reference in her case notes concerning the birth. The very nature of sexual violence made the gathering of source material extremely difficult.[30] Not only was it a taboo subject, but the abuse took place behind closed doors and only came to light in very rare cases, such as when a woman became pregnant. Abused women were often naive or at least treated like children and because of this it was unlikely that they would have been believed if they made accusations against the men who were supposed to be responsible for their well-being and safety. The religious ambiance of the nineteenth century further obscured the records, as women who were seduced or even raped were seen as having 'fallen from grace'.

Records of women in the County Cork Mental Asylum in Ireland contained strong implications that abuse was taking place in the female wards.[31] One 46-year-old woman said that 'they' wanted to put her to hell because she was not 'made like other people'. She believed that Jack the Ripper, who was active between the years 1888–1891, came to her in the night and 'did something to her'. She had not been the same since. A twenty-year-old, single young woman was recorded as having delusions. Her case notes indicated that she had told the doctor that bad men came into the ward at night and had sex with some of the female patients. The young woman could not sleep because she was in dread that they might come to her whilst going from bed to bed.

Victorian society's attitude towards disturbed and ill females affected the manner in which they were cared for. This can be seen in the case of Emily Moore from the East End of London. Born in 1847 she received a basic education and at the age of ten developed epilepsy. The condition was supposed to have been brought about by her receiving a sudden shock when her brother-in-law frightened her, entering the room wearing a sheet. Following her first 'attack', Emily was placed in Bethnal Green mental asylum. Despite her illness, Emily became a servant but was still subject to fits, which made her very distressed. She 'lamented her condition to a friend' whose response was that if she were 'so afflicted' she would drown herself. In 1866 Emily followed her friend's advice and attempted suicide by drowning. She was admitted to the City of London Mental Asylum where she was diagnosed as suffering from 'melancholia with epilepsy'. Her condition was 'unchanged' until 19 May 1869 when, at the age of twenty-two, she gave birth to a baby boy within the 'safe' environs of the asylum; the baby was removed from her immediately. She recovered from the confinement but was noted as suffering from milk retention as she was not allowed to nurse her child. There was no explanation as to how or by whom Emily became pregnant. Three years later, at the age of twenty-five, Emily died in the asylum. This account of what, with hindsight, was a case of mental and physical abuse of a vulnerable, young woman was made possible largely due to the prevailing attitudes towards females in general. The way in which Emily was treated in the asylum suggested that she was held responsible for her depression, her suicidal thoughts and her susceptibility to predatory men. This was borne out by the fact that she was punished by having her baby taken away from her before it was weaned, even though that made her physically ill, following the common treatment meted out to unmarried mothers. The unpleasant reality that women were not safe from sexual abusers, even in mental asylums, can be observed in the scant records of these institutions.

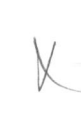

Some private lunatic asylums appear to have been no better than the county ones or Ireland's County Cork. Private lunatic asylums in Bethnal Green and Hoxton were owned by proprietor Thomas Warburton who became infamous for running ill-managed and brutal establishments. The journalist John Mitford, who spent some time in the Hoxton Asylum, petitioned Parliament unsuccessfully to investigate the conditions in these madhouses. Although Mitford had been denigrated as a sensational hack, one who certainly had issues with Thomas Warburton and his asylums, he reflected Victorian ideas and perceptions around madness and asylums. Through exposing 'true' stories, in which the victims were identified, he was able to show the dangers posed by unregulated and uncontrolled keepers. His history of Thomas Warburton brought the Victorian reader's attention to the abuse within the walls of private asylums:

> Thomas Warburton Esq. Keeper of the asylums for lunatics, Whitmore House, Hoxton – Mare Street, Hackney – Bethnal Green – and several minor establishments in Kingsland Road, & etc. & etc., was originally a butcher's boy in the country, and fled to London before he had served the term of his apprenticeship, for having a bastard child swore to him. He was first employed under the porter at the gate of Whitmore House, to beat coats, clean shoes and carry messages, for which he was rewarded with his meat. Being expert in conveying liquor into the house for the keepers to dispose of amongst their patients (a practice still pursued) he obtained a footing as a servant, and in that situation, by a little help and much industry, he learned to read and write. His strength of body (a necessary qualification for a demon in one of those hells) and his zeal, raised him to the dignity of a keeper, and he assumed controul of the lash under happy auspices. He is more than six foot high, broad shoulders, heavy built, with knock knees and a visage on which there is a proboscis three inches long, quite sufficient to frighten a person of weak mind and delicate nerves into a fit of insanity. ... In time he attained the confidential office of first keeper and by his treatment

of the lunatics under his care, gained the good graces of his mistress, who, upon the death of her husband, married him and he became the ruler over the mansion of affliction.[32]

In documenting Warburton's low birth and shady past, Mitford highlighted how inappropriate he was to be in charge of mental patients, especially the female ones. His low class was an important factor, as the relatives of most of the patients would not want to place their family members at the mercy of an illiterate ex-butcher boy with dubious, sexual morals. Among the male and female keepers in Warburton's asylum, whom he described as 'rogues and prostitutes',[33] he singled out one, an especially rough and violent man, Peter Parker and his 'Atrocious cases of violation … of three insane females':

> This monster, Peter Parker, is the house-carpenter and occasionally gives assistance as a keeper; his office as carpenter, at various times, gives him access to every part of this prison house, amongst his brothers in iniquity, who, no doubt, are equally guilty, but less known. He is a sort of 'Lothario', a braggart who boasts of his triumph over helpless women, whom I should deem it worse than death to look upon with any eyes but those of pity, and think it sacrilege to touch, but with a protecting hand.

Mitford accused Parker of rape:

> Ann Baldwin was a patient of a very tender age and had she been in her perfect health and senses, quite incapable of resisting the brutal assaults of such a fellow as Parker, but she had not a spark of reason at any time to direct her ways, and was, no doubt, a passive victim in the villain's hands. She became pregnant and brought forth a child of misery, destined never to be recognised by its mother, and if it lives, must abhor its father.[34]

Warburton allowed Parker to keep his post as keeper, even when he found out what had been going on in his asylum. This shocked Mitford, who also blamed Parker for the pregnancies of several young patents, including Martha Jones, a 'wretched maniac', and Ellen, a victim of his 'brutal lust'. He was incensed by the notion that predatory males were permitted to abuse defenceless inmates of private lunatic asylums. In Victorian England, other institutions, convents in particular, were seen as places of danger for young girls[35] and anti-Catholic writers would stir the moral conscience of British men by stressing how helpless females were easy prey for unscrupulous priests. By creating for himself, a persona who was the defender of some of the most vulnerable women in England, Mitford was able to make a strong and sensational case against these asylums and strike fear into the hearts of his readers.

One of the patients in the Hoxton asylum was Miss Rolleston,[36] who was the daughter of Stephen Rolleston, chief clerk in the Secretary of State's office. Mitford described her as an amiable and interesting girl who had already been in the asylum for some time before he met her. According to Mitford, the young lady's parents were very anxious about her recovery. She had, at intervals, 'dawnings of reason' and at such times she was admitted to the parlour where she conducted herself in such a becoming way that he was convinced that 'kind treatment would have restored her to her afflicted parents *compos mentis*.' This belief was further endorsed by the fact that he had partnered Miss Rolleston at cards and they had won. However, two months after the card game she was in the garden and Mitford observed that she was 'nearly frantic, the indecency of her actions was deplorable'. He 'chanced to go out of the door' and witnessed Miss Rolleston's keeper, Mrs Radley, beating her with a broomstick on her breast. The young woman flew to Mitford and said: 'Won't you save me? You know we won at cards t'other night'. He protected her and took her safely to her room as he knew that neither Mr Warburton nor any of his agents, knowing who Mitford was, were inclined to say anything to upset or anger him. Of course this 'reporting' could be merely sensation, but the use of names and places would suggest otherwise, as would the efforts of 'The Alleged Lunatics' Friend Society'.[37]

Mitford was clearly upset that the Rollestons were under the illusion that their daughter was being well cared for. He remarked that they were 'of the highest state of affluence and they fondly hoped and foolishly believed that Mr Warburton could restore their lost child'; however, they were continually informed that she was worse than before. He did not mention whether he had informed the Mitfords of their daughter's treatment or if they had read his writing on the subject. It is not possible, therefore, to know why they let her remain in such an establishment. Mitford asserted that Miss Rolleston was being 'violated by the filthy dungeon villains inhabiting Mr Warburton's madhouse'. Apparently, a young man named Kelly slept in the same bed as Miss Rolleston many Saturday nights by the contrivance of Mrs Burning, the 'keepress of the gaol'. Mitford claimed that he had seen them in bed together at least twenty times. Even worse, he maintained that:

> I have seen the person of that child, for so I must call one bereft of reason, prostituted on the steps leading to the Lodge by more than one keeper. I have heard it mentioned to Warburton and his answer has been, 'it is of no matter; she don't know what is done to her.' I could not, at that time, take it upon me to knock the villain down who used such language, revolting to human nature; but thank Heaven, I live to record his infamy and make the world abhor him.[38]

Mitford said that there was something about Miss Rolleston that made him both love and pity the poor girl who was visited by 'the scourge of human darkness'. In his impassioned defence, he fell into nineteenth-century idiom when he described women as being gentle lambs at the mercy of the ravenous wolf and he ended his account by writing:

> Alas poor child of misery! Thy bosom has been rifled by villains; thy treasures were stolen and thy ways corrupted by monsters. Methinks I never saw a fairer form under middle size – but what avails form, or face, when the gate of desolation is opened and the ravenous wolf can prey upon the lamb without an eye to pity – an ear to hear – or a hand to defend.[39]

The women who were abused in Victorian asylums were frequently referred to as lambs. This was a direct reference from the book of the prophet Jeremiah in the Old Testament where he refers to being led like a gentle lamb to slaughter.[40] This pastoral image had, over time, taken on its own particular significance and would have been immediately recognizable to the biblically literate Victorians. It was generally accepted that if someone went like a lamb to the slaughter, they did it without knowing that something bad was going to happen to them. It followed, therefore, that they acted calmly without fighting against the situation. Whilst it is impossible for us to know how these young women dealt with their abuse, it was apparent that many of them believed that their sufferings were their own fault and that they were being punished by God for some sin they had committed. This thought process would have made them especially vulnerable to manipulative predators.

It was agreed, by all concerned with the welfare of female asylum patients, that they had to be protected against sexual abuse, particularly rape. In his book, *Lunacy: Its Past and Present,* (1870) Dr Robert Gardiner Hill asserted that during the first half of the nineteenth century, there were many cases of female asylum patients being made pregnant by male keepers or male patients. By the middle of the century security on the female wards was increased and at Colney Hatch, the doctors and the chaplains were the only men to have keys. When a breach of this security took place and a child was born in the hospital, the baby was immediately removed from its mother and handed over to her home parish or to the workhouse. As the county asylums became over-populated and in many cases developed into mere warehouses for the mad, the care of the patients deteriorated. Ever-increasing cost of running the asylums meant that the management could not afford to pay good wages to the keepers and nurses and so the calibre of those employed declined, leaving the female patients even more vulnerable to sexual exploitation.

Women with Religious Excitement

Yet still, from time to time, vague and forlorn
From the Soul's subterranean depth unborne
As from an infinitely distant land,
Come airs, and floating echoes, and convey
A melancholy into all our day.

From: Matthew Arnold, *The Buried Life* 1852

The hypothesis that 'religious excitement' was a gendered category in nineteenth-century mental health diagnosis is supported by the case notes of William Scott who was an inmate of Bethlem in 1855. William was a young man, fifteen years old, an apprentice to a compositor; however, age consideration did not seem to come into diagnosis. He spoke of having lived in places he had never been to, that he had frequently committed murder and often saw devils. He also believed that he had been hanged, was dead and that he saw devils and spirits around him. His notes read that his conduct was 'more like that of an hysterical girl than that of an insane person'. Nothing more was recorded about William Scott other than he was discharged 'cured' just three months after his admission, his hysteria gone. William was presumably deemed to be a masculine young man once more.

Writing on religion and insanity in 1909,[1] Dr Charles Williams pointed out that many members of the medical profession thought religion to be the cause of a good deal of the insanity prevailing in England. He thought this justified, since of the numerous persons who became insane every year and had to be transferred to asylums, a large proportion had religious delusions, or at least talked a great deal on the subject of religion. However, he surmised that it was not nearly so often responsible as would first appear. He cited an example of one of his patients. A young girl suddenly, one night, became 'raving mad'. Williams found her in a state of acute mania and all her ravings were on religion. One delusion she had was that she was the Virgin Mary. This went on for some days and she was moved to the county lunatic asylum where the cause of her madness was put down to religion. Later it transpired that the real cause of her lunacy was fright. On the night in question the girl had gone out on an errand and had become perturbed by the behaviour of some man. When the attack of insanity took hold of her, her delusions took a religious turn. Unfortunately, Williams did not go on to explain why a young girl who was traumatized by a man's behaviour should translate her fear into religious ravings. This, in itself, indicates the possible acceptance by doctors that religion was all-pervasive in Victorian society.

Dr George Savage, who was Physician Superintendent at Bethlem Royal Hospital until 1888, supported Williams in his initial theory. Known for his case-based approach to psychiatry, he held that religion was generally only a partial cause. He assessed that whilst it was true that religion often 'colours' insanity, the responsibility for actually causing it must nearly always be placed elsewhere. In his work on insanity and neuroses, Savage said:

> Probably few causes of insanity are more frequently in the mouth of the general public than religious excitement; and yet the experience of the asylum physician is that religious excitement does not produce any large proportion of the cases which come under his observation … There is a very great distinction to be made between the many cases which exhibit some religious symptoms and the few which are really caused by religion itself.[2]

Again we have the assertion that it was not actually religion that was causing the type of insanity which was diagnosed as 'religious excitement' or 'religious mania', simply that religion was a useful category given the symptoms. The type of religious education offered to girls, particularly working-class girls, offers insight as to why religion and madness were so closely linked.[3]

In another case, this time concerning a Baptist woman, it could be seen that following years of physical exhaustion and possibly mental upset, 56-year-old Catherine Watson finally experienced some kind of psychological meltdown which was so extreme and frightening that she could only express it in terms of having been 'affected by the Devil'. Biblical language was often used by women to express their despair. As we saw in the previous chapter, the loss of children frequently precipitated a woman's breakdown and therefore grief was displayed in religious terms.

Married to a coach wheelwright for thirty-four years when admitted to the Hanwell Asylum in 1857, Catherine was recorded as being delicate in health, nervous for the past six years and of a 'naturally excitable disposition'. She had given birth to eleven children but only two of them were alive. Her mental breakdown had started on her way home from chapel, when she had suddenly thrown up her arms and said, 'Now I see the Devil' and then exclaimed, 'Get thee behind me Satan'. She was said to be of a 'religious turn' and was in the habit of going to hear religious preachers. Since the Sunday in question her behaviour had been very different from usual and she had made violent attempts to confine her husband whom she locked in a room and threatened to kill. She was said to have raved constantly and chiefly on religion. Finally, we learnt that Catherine said that she saw the Saviour; she sang hymns and appeared elated in spirits.

Grief over the death of children was often expressed in 'religious excitement'. Catherine had lost nine children over a span of around twenty years, which must have affected her psychologically. Nor was it extraordinary that in some way she appeared to blame or hate her husband for her situation. The fact that she liked to go and hear different preachers pointed to the possibility that she was searching for some kind of alleviation from or reason for her suffering. Maybe, like Jane Peakes, she had heard something in the sermon that Sunday that resonated with her mental condition and produced a vision of the Devil. Whatever happened, that day she seemed to have found some consolation in Jesus to whom she was able to sing hymns which raised her spirits. Nothing more was recorded about Catherine's medical treatment, if any, or how her illness progressed. After a month in the asylum she was discharged.

Religious excitement and gender

Religious excitement or religious mania was often cited as an 'exciting' cause for the admission of a woman into a mental asylum during the nineteenth century and this frequently inappropriately named condition manifested itself in a particular way amongst the female patients. Despite the fact these terms were in common usage as descriptions of a patient's mental state, it is not altogether clear what exactly was meant by them and they seemed to indicate something different when applied to either men or women. Religion and religious language was used, markedly by women, to express feelings of inadequacy, lack of confidence in their own self-worth and abilities and notions of guilt and sin. This was different from the way in which males employed similar terminology. When men invoked God or the Devil they were usually justifying their actions, which were often aggressive.

An illustration of a woman suffering from religious excitement can be seen in the case of Martha Higgins who was admitted to the Hanwell Asylum in February 1846 from the workhouse at Hanover Square. Martha was a single woman who was acting so violently that she was admitted in a straight jacket, kicking. Once released from the restraint, she walked up and down the room, with an air of great delight and satisfaction, and did not attempt to molest anyone. She had been left an orphan, had 'been seduced' and had gone on to live a 'most dissolute' life in London. 'Drunkenness and debauch' were thought to have brought on the disease she was now suffering. She imagined herself the recipient of angels' visits, and she expressed herself towards them in terms of rapture and devotion. Her 'religious delusions' continued to be commented on and it became clear that she was physically ill as well as mentally disturbed. This was a common occurrence in the notes of female mental patients which often read as if the physical condition was merely coincidental. Martha exhibited eccentric conduct which was dependent on her religious hallucinations. She had exhibited no great amount of violent conduct since the day of her admission and had not required a moment's 'seclusion'. 'Seclusion' was intended to reduce the possibility of patients behaving in a violent and destructive way. They were removed from the ward and left alone in a, frequently darkened, room. Dr John Conolly who, in 1856, argued in favour of the abolishment of mechanical restraints in the treatment of asylum, advocated the use of seclusion for those violent patients whose exclusion from external stimuli was considered to be therapeutic.

From the mid-nineteenth century, asylums used the 'padded room' or 'cell' to isolate patients. These rooms were custom-built, constructed with strong, waterproof ticking stuffed with cocoa-nut fibre or horse hair; even the floors were padded, covered with thick mattresses. However, a warm bath and the nightly use of a sedative with a mild aperient draught to relieve constipation appeared to have been beneficial to Martha. She complained about much aching about the 'limbs' and was suffering from 'leucorrhoeal discharge' from the vagina for which she was being treated. This is a yellow or white discharge that can be an indication of infection or sexually transmitted disease. Martha's 'story' developed in a manner that blamed her illness on her sexual behaviour. Her religious delusions were inextricably linked to her mental state which was caused by a sense of sin.

A month after Martha's admittance she was transferred to 'the quiet ward' as she was no longer violent. Although her delusions respecting angels and glories visibly surrounding her continued, her conduct was subdued and tranquil. As her religious delusions continued, her health deteriorated. Finally, Martha was removed to the infirmary in consequence of her complaining of increased weakness accompanied by a continuous discharge from her vagina. Her mind was now more calm, and she was beginning to distinguish between the impressions of her own brain and the things of sense around her. In other words, Martha now recognized that the 'visions' and 'glories' which surrounded her were not real but due to her state of health which improved enough for the doctor to report, 'Miss H has refrained from an allusion to the phantoms which occupied her when she was first admitted' and, 'the mucus discharge has in a great deal subsided and her general health is much improved.' If, as suggested above, Martha's vaginal discharge was a symptom of venereal disease, there was no mention of any specific treatment apart from warm baths. It was known that syphilis could cause insanity so presumably it was not suspected. If another sexually transmitted disease, like gonorrhoea, had been diagnosed as the result of her immoral behaviour, her feelings of guilt and sin, together with her weakened, physical state would have been the most likely causes of her insanity.

Another month passed and Martha's continued to improve. She was cheerful and kept herself occupied knitting and reading. She met with the chaplain and told him that she was sorry for her past life; however, she became distressed and tearful when he said that she might have avoided the reprobate life she pursued. Martha refused to talk any more about her past because she believed that she had not been given enough 'allowance' for the 'forlorn situation' she had found herself in and the temptations that she had faced. She took to reading the prayer book of the Church of England and the Bible daily, and her morbid fancies lessened. She was liberally supplied with books on practical religion and moral subjects by the chaplain, who had been advised by Martha's doctors to avoid giving her anything of an 'exciting doctrinal character'. Her physical health became better and her mental health stabilized to the extent that, five months after her admission, Martha Higgins was discharged from Hanwell, deemed cured.

The links between Martha's physical illness and her mental one could be traced through scanty medical records. However, why, as a sinner according to her, was she visited by angels and glories?[4] In his history of insanity, Michel Foucault asserted that the asylum was a religious domain without religion, that religion provoked madness because it excited a fear of the 'Beyond', which, in return, conjured up fearful images and strong emotions. These often led to despair and melancholia.[5] If religion provoked madness, then logically, the language of religion could be used to explain the fears and emotions that were caused by mental ill health and trauma. In this way, religious terminology was used as a kind of code for Victorian patients to vocalize their feelings.

Religious fervour came in different forms. Unlike Martha Higgins who saw her visions in terms of angels, Susannah Darman was faced with hallucinations of the Devil. Susannah was admitted to Hanwell Asylum in 1858 suffering from some kind of mental breakdown brought on by religion. The letter from her employer, which explained the situation to the superintendent, read as follows and showed a kind concern for his servant. It is worth quoting fully as it provides a picture of the negative influence religion could have on a gullible, young woman:

Dear Sir,

In December 1856 Susannah Darman entered my service as housemaid. She had a good character (from her last place in the country) and while here she has conducted herself to the entire satisfaction of her mistress except that she was slow in her work.

I attribute her present state solely to the fact that in January last under the influence of an exciting sermon at a Wesleyan chapel she was led the same evening to enroll her name as a member of that denomination, and on further reflection feeling that she had taken a step which ought to have been preceded by a larger knowledge of scripture than she then possessed she has since endeavoured to the best of her ability to study the New Testament but unfortunately the proceedings at these meetings she attended were more calculated to excite than to instruct and her mind became more and more perplexed until at last it has affected her reason.

During the last two or three weeks we were aware that her mind was perplexed and her mistress and my daughters frequently conversed with her on the subject but without any beneficial result, and on two or three occasions when I conversed with her myself I found she was endeavouring to understand the most difficult portion of the Revelations.

It was not until Wednesday last that we observed any indications that her mind was affected altho from what we have since learnt from her fellow servants it had probably been coming on for a few days previously. On Thursday morning at 3 am I was called up and found her very excited under the impression that the Devil was in the room, after a time she was calmed and retired again to bed and slept for three or four hours. Later in the morning she became more excited and about noon indications that her reason was affected were perceived, and in the afternoon she was removed.

I understand that since then she has spoken of a policeman or as to lend to an impression that that it was a love affair – but this I can explain by stating that a few weeks since there was a robbery committed in my warehouse and that the constable employed having called first in uniform, then in a rough dress, and afterwards dressed as a gentleman, so surprised her that she made it a subject of conversation.

Since her removal a copy of the Rules of the Wesleyans has been found and upon reading them I can clearly see that the poor girl took these in their most literal meaning and was endeavouring strictly to obey them. In my mind there is no doubt that her affliction is solely to be attributed to her endeavouring to obey rules the meaning of which were not explained to her and to understand difficult questions beyond her comprehension.

It may be right to state that her health has been good, and that she has not been subject to fits, and I am informed that none of her relations have been inflicted with insanity.

I shall be obliged (should you have the opportunity) by the attention of the chaplain of the asylum being requested to her case. Until January last she attended the services of the Church of England, and I should be glad if her attention could be fixed to the plain and simple truths of the Gospel.

Myself and family feel more interest in this case from the fact that she has neither father nor mother, or (to our knowledge) any relation who is able to take charge of her permanently we shall therefore be glad to be made acquainted with any change that may take place, and especially should there be a probability of her death, preceded by an interval of reason, I should be obliged by the earliest intimation of it.

With our thanks to Mrs. Davies and yourself for the kind attention you have shown this case.

I remain Dear Sir,
Yours faithfully,

James Bigg[6]

This letter was moving for the paternal care an employer might show for his female house servant; and enlightening in the way in which it reflected the current thinking on the danger of too much religious study and enthusiasm. The young woman was said to be an orphan and a maid in Mr Bigg's household and as such, her employer showed obvious concern for her, asking to be contacted if she should be in danger of dying, if she was able to communicate in sound mind. There was no mention of the possibility of her being cured and what would happen to her in the case of that eventuality.

Protestant enthusiasm

In his book on insanity (1838) Sir W.C. Ellis, the superintendent of the Asylum at Wakefield, gave an explanation of the term 'Religious Excitement' as a cause of madness. He stated: 'Too intense thought upon religious subjects is the moral cause, which, next to distressed circumstances and grief, has produced, as far as we have been able to ascertain, the greatest number of cases in the institution at Wakefield.'[7] He went on to say that he had found that this was a particularly English phenomenon: 'Very few of the patients in the asylums on the Continent are said to have become insane from this cause,'[8] something which he attributed to the fact that in some countries religious discussion was forbidden due to political reasons and in others it never took place due to 'the general prevalence of infidelity amongst the higher orders, and ignorance and blind superstitious obedience to the dictum of the priests amongst the lower classes'.[9] The other reason he gave for the high numbers of inmates suffering with Religious Excitement was very much in keeping with Mr Bigg's 'diagnosis' of his housemaid's condition:

> As there are more sectarians of all kinds in England than in any other part of the world except America, religion is more immediately brought home to the poor as a subject of thought and examination. Wherever a variety of opinion exists, and freedom of discussion is allowed, the attention is naturally roused, and the feelings become excited. And when the immortality of the soul, and the awful realities of eternity are first impressed upon the mind of an individual, who has never before given the subject any serious thought, he is led to consider those objects which he formerly pursued with avidity as altogether vain and delusive, and to devote the whole of his time and every mental energy, exclusively to the investigation of this now all-absorbing subject. When he finds that his conduct has to himself the awful; denunciations of Scripture, without receiving the consolations of its promises; the anticipation of that eternal misery, which he fancies to be his inevitable doom, continually fills his mind with gloomy apprehensions, and eventually sinks him into the most suffering state of insanity, from the over action of the brain in thinking of this subject.[10]

Ellis believed that it was dangerous for the uneducated classes to think or read too much, especially on religious subjects. In the nineteenth century, women were believed to be at risk from overstimulation of their brains; Susannah Darman would have been seen to be doubly vulnerable to new and provoking ideas presented by the Wesleyans as she was both uneducated and female.

Writing on insanity in 1844, A.L. Wiggins was in agreement with Ellis about the rarity of religious madness in Catholic countries. He attributed this to the practices of the Protestant clergy:

> Some Protestant clergymen, when first made acquainted with the doubts and embarrassments of their young and fragile-minded communicants, enter into explanatory discussions, recommend the study of the Bible and of works of theological controversy. The patient, at an age when the brain

is expanding perhaps faster than its bony covering can make room for growth, enters upon the investigation of subjects so abstruse that they have disturbed the intellect of the most able and energetic men. The poor girl (for it is most frequently, though by no means exclusively, in that sex that these doubts and delusions take root) becomes more and more bewildered. If it be only one of the brains in which the disease is beginning, the sound one, instead of performing its duty as a sentinel and controller, is taught to dwell constantly on the same morbid train of thoughts which occupy its fellow, and thus confirmed insanity is established, where a different mode of treatment would perhaps have restored the disordered brain to a healthy state.[11]

Wiggins pointed out that the practice of the Catholic clergy was exactly the opposite to the above, and he described their methods and the results they produced. He said that Catholic priests gave their communicants a large quantity of ceremonial devotion to perform and prayers to be recited and forbade all controversial or doctrinal reading. The incessant repetition of these prayers and observances had the soothing effect of all monotony and tranquilized the morbid emotions of the brain. He commented, from his own experience, that:

> It is also a principle with the Catholic clergy to confine the study of theology to themselves and entirely to discourage it in the laity. Thus one large source of mental disturbance is superseded. I have sometimes wished, when hearing flippant young girls discussing the abstruse doctrines and mysteries of religion, that a similar practice prevailed in our church with the young. I cannot shut my eyes as a medical man to the mischievous consequences of such studies to every brain whose delicate structure tends to insanity, nor to the advantage (medically speaking) of a system which puts such brains in repose.[12]

'Mad doctors' such as Wiggins did not dispute the belief that the influence of religion, of a 'tranquilizing faith', on the mental health of society was a good thing. However, he believed that religious mania was mainly caused by the uses of the religious sects and not by their theological tenets. He gave the following illustration to explain his theory:

> How many examples have I seen of innocent and virtuous girls who, if intended for nuns, would have been cured during their novitiate and would have returned to the world to become happy and respected mothers of families – how many such have I seen injudiciously encouraged to

pass their time in studying the mysteries of sanctification, regeneration, redemption, till they have rapidly progressed into positively insanity, and taken refuge from intolerable terrors in suicide. How often have I felt anguish of the heart at witnessing these horrors and being utterly unable to prevent them. I have heard these pure and innocent creatures accuse themselves of impossible crimes, and die in the agonies of despair, while the bystanders attributed the unnatural accusations to remorse at having ceded to the instigations of the devil.[13]

The case of Susannah Darman combined elements of low class and lack of education with religious fervour and it is salient that all three were seen as contributing to women's madness. As previously mentioned, Susannah was completely alone in the world, no parents, no relatives. There was mention of a possible love interest, a policeman who was employed by Mr Bigg to investigate a robbery at his warehouse. This liaison was dismissed by her employer, presumably as a fantasy. However, a lonely girl in a house where there were daughters, possibly of a similar age, might have felt her position very acutely. Being a country girl not used to London ways, Susannah may well have misinterpreted the policeman and read a friendly dalliance as a love affair. The fact that Susannah immersed herself in religion would seem to be more like a symptom of her condition rather than its cause. Her overstudy of scripture and vulnerability to dramatic proselytising preachers, which resulted in her obsessive behaviour, was seen by her master as the origin of her breakdown. Over-study, especially of religious doctrine, was seen as a cause of madness especially for a female of Susannah's class and education who would be deemed unable to understand fully what she was reading.

The loneliness of the single, working woman

The problems experienced by young women who were sent away from home to work in other people's houses as servants or even governesses filled the pages of Victorian novels as well as the casebooks of Victorian asylums. In the nineteenth century, domestic service was the largest occupation of women. Young, unmarried girls sent into service as young as thirteen were employed as maids-of-all-work, general servants, to carry out the most menial chores. Susannah Darman was described by her employer as a 'housemaid', which meant that she had been hired to work 'above stairs' rather than in the kitchen or scullery. In middle- and upper-class families, the servants lived in. Susannah's previous place had been 'in the country' so she would have been without friends and family in London. However kind her employer and family were, she would have been considered to have been on a different level from them and treated accordingly.

Another single servant was 24-year-old Jane Peakes, a patient in Bethlem from December 1857 to December 1858 suffering from 'religious enthusiasm'. She supposedly became 'very much excited after a sermon one Sunday in the hospital chapel', which resulted in her becoming suicidal and delusional and 'the loss of the menses'. She spent a year in Bethlem before being discharged, 'cured'. Against a background of this prevailing theory about religious excitement, a suicidal young girl was diagnosed with a condition that was brought on by the 'over-study of religion'. Jane believed that her Aunt and Uncle would die unless she herself did. A closer reading of her notes would suggest that Jane was suffering from delusions and whilst she was listening to the hospital chaplain preach she declared that he had made a reference to her and her spiritual condition. At this time Bethlem was noted for giving patients decent food and rest, which may have been exactly what this young woman needed. Possibly it was that simple treatment that led to her being cured. The catamenia reappeared after several months in the asylum but she 'remained childish'.

The number of women who struggled under the illusion that their condition was a deserved punishment for breaking some rule of religion suggests that they were frequently placed into hallowed roles they could not fulfil. Wesleyan spinster, 27-year-old Sarah Culmer Dadds believed that she was 'lost forever and was perishing fast', when she was admitted to Bethlem Hospital in June 1856. Sarah worked as a governess with a family when the first symptoms manifested and in consequence she was obliged to leave her post. When initially in Bethlem, her health deteriorated and it was recorded that she had 'unpleasant habits'. This description was usually a veiled a reference to masturbation, but it could also have signified the distasteful way in which she picked nervously at her skin, a sign of anxiety and a form of self-harm. Sarah was seriously depressed and believed that her life had 'passed away', that she was dying. Physically unhealthy, constipated, thin and much disfigured by sores exacerbated by picking, her hands and nails were almost deprived of cuticles and other parts of her body were in a poor state. Her claims that she had 'sinned grievously' and was 'perishing' and 'sinking into hell' were accompanied by 'lamentations' and 'much weeping'. Sarah's state of mental wretchedness rendered her sufferings unbearable and prevented sleep, and it was feared that she would die of exhaustion. However, after being given 'morphia and food of a nourishing character', the symptoms somewhat abated. She contentedly drank the wine, porter given to her, and, although the delusions continued, the mental anguish diminished. The next observation to be written down was that her health had improved and four months after her admission she was discharged 'cured', presumably her religious delusions had disappeared as she became physically stronger.

Again, this scanty case history, which was fairly typical, fails to provide reasons as to why and how certain outcomes were arrived at. The treatment given to the patients was poorly recorded and the reason for their admission to an asylum can only be assumed. Sarah's case of severe depression was shared by many governesses. Her education provided no protection against the deprivations she suffered due to her position and class. Sarah reverted to the only explanation she could think of for her illness, that she was being punished for her sins. Unlike Susannah Darman, who had a decent employer in Mr Bigg, Sarah had to leave her employment so presumably it would have been almost impossible for her to find another post.

Even educated women attributed their melancholia or suicidal feelings to religion. Like Sarah Culmer Dadds, Emma Austen was a single governess. Her attack of insanity, when she was thirty-one, was said to have originated in gastric fever and over-exertion. She became suicidal and it was noted that her sister was similarly affected. Emma's two certificates of admission stated that she had a 'morbid and melancholy appearance' and she said that she had 'lost her soul and that God would not forgive her'. Emma said that she was 'not alive', had no feeling and was not like anyone else. She thought that she was 'drawing others to perdition by mixing with them or even by shaking hands with them'. She was constantly melancholy, did not want to eat at times and had attempted suicide. Emma was said to have 'delusions as to the destruction of her soul', thinking that it was a sin to destroy the body as in so doing the soul was destroyed. She charged herself with crimes for which there were no grounds. Her doctor believed that she intended to commit suicide and this had to be guarded against as she had 'every symptom of lunacy'. It was noted that she had had an illness whilst she was living in Hastings, which she said that she feigned and had deceived everybody. She was initially pale and thin, but whilst in the asylum she began to eat well. She was portrayed as being very clean and tidy, particularly about her appearance. Her notes said that she was very good with the other patients and as her depression lifted and her delusions faded, she became positively amiable and chatty. Tragically, Emma had been misdiagnosed and she died of pulmonary tuberculosis.

The job of governess was one particular female occupation that was recognized by nineteenth-century doctors of the mind as being particularly detrimental to mental health. Dr George Savage, who was the superintendent and physician of Bethlem, a lecturer on mental diseases at Guys Hospital and the co-editor of *The Journal of Medical Science*, wrote the following after commenting on the large number of governesses in Bethlem: 'To my mind the governess's life is a very good example of the predisposing causes of insanity.'[14] Sisters Ann and Charlotte Brontë understood the serious emotional constraints put upon governesses and how this very solitary occupation could lead to mental breakdown. The combination of overwork, loneliness and ill health with a sense of abandonment by God and self-deprecation can be found in nineteenth-century novels. In *Villette* by Charlotte Brontë, the heroine, Lucy Snowe, suffers a mental breakdown when she is left alone during the school vacation. Her state of mind, brought on by her extreme loneliness, forces her to enter a Catholic church and make a confession. In the confessional, Lucy finds a hidden space where she can admit what is really troubling her. Whilst she is in the church, Lucy watches the penitents going to confession and her perception is that they are all women receiving consolation, something that she needed badly. Brontë herself understood the consolation of confession from her own experiences of loneliness and despair when she was left alone at the Pensionnat Heger in Brussels during the long Summer vacation of 1843 and when she, like Lucy Snowe, knelt at the confessional in St. Gudule's Cathedral.[15] It would seem that both author and heroine used the confessional more as a psychiatrist's couch than as a channel for the forgiveness of their sins.

By the mid-1850s there had been a sharp rise in the number of families employing a governess to teach and take care of their children. The 1851 census showed that 25,000 women were working as governesses in England. Governesses and teachers in small, private, girls' schools very often came from gentile poverty, being the daughters of the clergy or middle-class fathers who had fallen on hard times. From the beginning of the nineteenth century the upper-middle classes began to copy their wealthier counterparts and employed governesses for their daughters and young sons. These women were sometimes from a superior class to their employers and yet were treated as somebody who was higher than a domestic servant but lower than the family with whom they lived. The governess was responsible not only for giving the children a basic education but was also charged with the children's moral instruction. They were often disliked by the household servants as they were supposed to be treated with respect even though they were working women. Governesses were notoriously badly paid, having very little salary over and above their board and lodging; they were therefore unable to save for their old age and this could lead to mental and physical breakdown in young women. As mentioned in the article on the modern governess system in *Fraser's Magazine* (1844), the statistics touching lunatic asylums gave a frightful proportion of governesses in the list of the insane.

Nineteenth-century England was difficult for a single woman. Although her allotted goal and frequent destiny were to be married and have children, according to the 1851 census there were over 365,000 more women than men in the country. This statistic meant that there were large numbers of women who could never even hope to become wives and mothers and was especially true for middle class, 'penniless' girls. These educated young women had very few professions open to them apart from teaching and even this work, being outside the home, meant that they would lose some of their social status creating a situation that often broke their spirit.

Unlike Susannah Darman and Jane Peakes, Emma Austen had received a good education and would have been of higher social standing. As is well documented, particularly by such writers as Charlotte and Anne Brontë, the governess played a very difficult role in the household; she was neither servant nor family and was frequently held in contempt by those above and beneath her. This led to isolation and loneliness. Governesses were also known to suffer from malnutrition, which, together with overwork, made them vulnerable to bodily as well as mental illness. Even though her physical illness had not been recognized, Emma would have benefitted from Bethlem's regime of good food, rest and useful occupation.

Religion and its effects on vulnerable women

Mental disturbance is both frightening and incomprehensible and sufferers often struggle to find a language that can even begin to express what they are feeling. Modern psychological jargon had not yet been invented in the nineteenth century which was an era seeped in religion and religious controversy; consequently, Victorian women frequently described their symptoms in religious terminology. Even those with the most basic of educations would have studied the Bible, and, from an early age, churchgoing was an important communal and religious activity. For both the middle and lower classes, social life revolved around church services and activities. Many employers insisted that their employees went to church and Sunday became an important day for leaving the house and meeting other people in the locality as well as listening to the weekly sermon. The language of religion, of heaven, hell, sin and forgiveness was present in everyday parlance. With divisions of the church, a new style of preaching became popular and had an evident influence on some impressionable women. In 1738, John Wesley had founded the Methodist Church and during the nineteenth century there was a revival of religious fervour. Under the designation of non-conformism, other breakaway sects from the Anglican Church emerged as evangelizing movements and their style of proselytizing had an obvious effect on many women. The main denominations being Baptists, Congregationalists, Presbyterians and Methodists.

The Baptists seem to have been responsible for influencing many women,[16] such as Elizabeth Ashdown, a single woman 'of the Baptist persuasion' admitted to Bethlem in 1859 after feeling suicidal and presenting as a danger to others. In her case, her doctors assessed her state of mind to be 'excited by religion'. She believed that everybody around her was wicked, but 'none so much as herself'. Elizabeth said that she had done something she could not reveal and 'she could never be forgiven'. She believed that she was constantly under surveillance and that even the people with their night-lights on in their bedrooms were keeping watch over her. This delusion pointed to her suffering from insomnia as she could see the night lights in the houses around her. The inability to sleep was recognized as a symptom of insanity, in particular, melancholia. Writing in 1868, Henry Maudsley observed:

> There is usually a great want of sleep, although patients are apt to assert that they have not slept when they really have, so little has been the feeling of refreshment therefrom. They are often tormented by vivid or painful dreams, their delusions pursuing them in their restless and unrefreshing slumbers.[17]

Elizabeth said that she 'must do murder', but that at present she lacked the courage to do it to herself, her mother or her sister. Another factor thought to contribute to her insanity was heredity; her mother had attempted to cut her own throat some years before. At one stage, Elizabeth had taken up a knife and placed it on her throat saying, 'I only wish I had the moral courage'. She claimed that she had something on her mind and 'only God knew how it would terminate'. She was convinced that she has sinned beyond redemption, and although she had always been morbidly strict in the observance of her religion, she had not been to any place of worship in the last six months in order to say her prayers, because she believed that it would be an offence for her to do so. The doctors diagnosed her as 'greatly depressed in mind, melancholic with delusions on religious subjects and having suspicions about food'. They remarked that she was a person of the Baptist persuasion who had devoted her whole time to the study of religious matters, which would indicate that they thought her affiliation with the Baptist church had some influence on her current state of mind. This was buttressed by her friends who told them that this over-studying had detrimentally affected her mind and had given rise to her symptoms of insanity, resulting in acute melancholia and 'a troublesome eruption on the face'. The doctor noted that 'the catamenia have appeared only twice during the last twelve months' meaning that her periods were irregular and had nearly ceased. This begs the question whether Elizabeth was experiencing an early menopause given her age (forty-eight). She was discharged from Bethlem in April 1859, 'uncured' and 'despairing in tears'. The doctors evidently felt that they could not do anything more to help Elizabeth and so she had to leave. Bethlem was essentially a 'curative establishment' and by its foundation was limited to curable cases unlike the county asylums. Elizabeth could have been discharged into the workhouse, a private or county asylum or to the care of her friends and family.

Delusions originating in biblical stories of Moses and Elijah in the Old Testament and the temptations of Jesus in the New Testament distressed 61-year-old Mary Ann Angell, the wife of a hairdresser and the mother of eleven children, who imagined that she had been commanded by God to 'abstain from eating food' and to pass the remainder of her days amongst wild animals in a state of complete nudity. Like the prophets before him, Jesus went out into the desert where he fasted for forty days and forty nights. As Mary Ann was fearful of being thought of as a 'drunkard and a glutton' and was visited by 'friends of the Devil' who had enslaved her, she felt the need for penance. After four months in Bethlem, Mary died from 'exhaustion followed by acute melancholia'. From the scant notes on Mary's condition and the contributing causes it is impossible to know what was really wrong with her. However, a woman of her age and social standing must have been physically and mentally exhausted after giving birth to and rearing eleven children. Postmenopausal and with her youngest child now eighteen, she was looking into a difficult old age. She had decided, at this point in her life, to 'deny her husband', meaning that she refused to have sex with him, and this was seen as a symptom of her madness. Mary Ann could use the excuse that she was being commanded by God to stop eating and avoid having sex with her husband and she was under the power of the Devil as a way of expressing her mental turmoil.

Women incarcerated in mental hospitals experienced an overwhelming feeling that God had abandoned them or was punishing them. They used a specifically gendered interpretation of their own mental state which relied on their belief that their affliction was the result of some past sin. While men too heard voices from God and believed that they had transgressed, women believed that they deserved some sort of retribution.

Religious excitement, sin and suffering

Forty-one reissues of Robert Burton's *Anatomy of Melancholy* (1621),[18] notable for its explanation of religious melancholy and mental health, were published in the nineteenth century. The third section of *The Anatomy* dealt with two aspects of melancholy as Burton perceived them. These were 'love melancholy' or love sickness and 'religious melancholy', which, either by its causes or symptoms, was associated with religion. Burton's treatise on religious melancholy was something new for its time; he had no pattern to follow because no physician had ever written about it. He believed that both the cause and the effect of this illness were often of a religious character and he recognized that the inordinately pious were highly susceptible. He backed up this theory by observing that self-mortification, solitude and long continued meditation on questions of faith engendered the melancholy humour. This in turn affected the fantasy and misled the intellectual faculty. Immoderate fasting, bad diet, sickness, melancholy and solitariness debilitated the sufferer and made them believe that Devil was controlling them. The form of religious melancholy that interested Burton most was an excruciating diffidence. Patients developed a morbid consciousness of their wickedness, forgot the all-embracing love and mercy of God and despaired of salvation. He acknowledged that, according to his beliefs, there were those whose affliction of conscience was rationally grounded, and these were those whose sins actually warranted a fear of damnation. However, Burton was concerned only with those whose despair was due to pathological fears and melancholy. He thought that too much religiosity engendered this melancholy and melancholy engendered fear in a vicious cycle. The patient therefore developed the delusion that his or her transgressions were beyond forgiveness. Many were terrified by imaginary demons and hellfire and were often driven to blasphemy and self-harming.

Burton's ideas fitted with those of the nineteenth-century mad doctors. However, according to the records of so many women incarcerated in asylums with a diagnosis of religious melancholy or mania, their condition was not often 'excited' by excessive fasting, solitary meditation on religious questions or self-mortification as he suggested. An example can be seen in Fanny Smith[19] who was admitted to the Colney Hatch Asylum in 1894, suffering from religious mania and hearing voices. She experienced the kitchen floor rising up and the houses in the street leaning as if they were about to fall over and she understood these as signs of the end of the world when she would be punished for her sins. Her mother told her that these premonitions were delusions, but Fanny believed them to be true and that she was under some punishment because a woman had told her that she was a heretic. Fanny cried and said that she could see people dying in flames, apparently a vision of Hell. As Church of England, she would have been informed of the idea of purgatory and the flames of Hades as the eternal retribution for sinners. Her mother informed the doctors that Fanny started asking strange religious questions like 'When was the Messiah coming?' The evangelical wing of the Church of England held that the second coming of Christ, as predicted in the Bible, was imminent. Fanny may have been frightened by sermon or story that told her to be sure that she was free from sin when Jesus returned. She would suddenly kneel down and pray at any time, even when she was working, and she maintained that she had done something so wicked that she could not go to church. As with other cases, no mention was made of what sins Fanny thought she had committed.

Some women, however, were explicit about the sins they thought they were guilty of. Another single, servant, nineteen-year-old Ellen Roche, entered Colney Hatch that same year, with very specific notions about her sins, believing that she had 'killed thousands of people'. When asked how she had done this she replied, 'I became a woman in 1889, I have killed doctors, send for the priest'. Her employer said that Ellen kept crying and screaming and threatening to cut her own throat. In 1889, Ellen was fourteen and her statement possibly alluded to beginning her periods, which were known in contemporary terms as 'the curse of Eve' following God's punishment of Eve in the Garden of Eden (Genesis 3:16-17). More likely, she was alluding to losing her virginity and had carried the guilt of being a 'sullied woman' with her ever since. Any woman in Victorian times who had sex before marriage would have been ostracized if the fact became common knowledge. Women were expected to remain virgins until they were married or their lives were threatened with ruin. Middle-class spinsters were supposed to help in the houses of parents or other relatives in return for economical support; however, they were not afforded the respect granted to wives and mothers. They were the ubiquitous 'maiden aunts', always second rate. Life was worse for unmarried working-class women who had to work in menial jobs without the help of a man's wage to support them. After nine months in the asylum, Ellen was discharged 'recovered'; it was not recorded if her employer took her back.

Many women admitted to Victorian asylums suffered from 'sub-acute melancholia' or 'religious melancholia' and had a deep sense of their own sin and unworthiness. Numerous patients suffering from depression were unable to pinpoint their actual misdemeanours, or were unwilling to say what they were, but they thought that they must have done something wrong in the eyes of God because they were being punished. Such distress could be observed in 25-year-old, Church of England, Elizabeth Thrussell, a fellow patient of Fanny and Ellen, also a single servant. She suffered from acute depression, 'weeping, moaning and wringing her hands whenever spoken to'. She ate very little, was restless and had 'a tendency to strip herself'. Elizabeth put her condition down to the fact that she had been very sinful and must suffer for her wickedness but could not describe the nature of her evil. Their inability to express their sinfulness may have been a lack of understanding of the church's espousal on sin, or, because they had been taught that suffering was the punishment for wickedness, they believed they must have done something bad to warrant their agony.

Twenty-six-year-old Rosa Mary Prattent, an earlier Hanwell patient (1847), suffered in a similar manner, said to be given to 'religious musings'. This member of the Church of England resorted to every kind of trick to obtain a prayer book or Bible, but whenever she succeeded in doing so she became much worse in her mind exclaiming throughout the night, 'My God, my God, why hast thou forsaken me?' This was the cry of torment uttered by Jesus at his crucifixion. The nurses were given strict injunctions to 'secure her from these sources of trouble and injury', in other words, to avoid giving her a Bible or prayer book. It was clear from her nocturnal crying that Rosa felt that she had been abandoned by God and she used the words from Jesus on the cross to express her psychological anguish. To this extent, Rosa was taking up Jesus's suffering, no doubt having been taught how we must all suffer to attain paradise.

Religion clearly haunted the mindset of the Victorian period. The importance of historical context to delusions has been written about by the twenty-first-century historian David Wright.[20] The way the afflicted attempted to articulate their suffering stems from the influences of Victorian society and the infusion of religion in everyday life. Female patients often found it difficult to express their feelings or describe traumatic events. With physical symptoms it was and is easier for the doctor to make a diagnosis and to evaluate the pain. Mental illness needed a new 'language' to convey what the patient was experiencing. The vocabulary of religion was accessible, natural and comprehensible to both the educated and the uneducated and was therefore a useful medium through which to explain fears, troubling emotions and sensations, even when those feelings arose from a perfectly understandable anxiety.

Grief was often the cause of serious mental distress. When thirty-five-year-old Maria Hine's husband was shipwrecked in 1849, she suffered a mental breakdown and was sent to the Hanwell Asylum where she remained 'insane' for a month suffering from what was referred to as 'religious delusions'; for example, she imagined that she had 'seen the Saviour crucified' and subsequently placed at a table near to hers'. She wept a lot, was despondent and had poor physical health, so stopped menstruating. This was the case with many women who had poor nutrition and ill health. In the asylum, Maria managed to get plenty of sleep and was given nourishing food, the usual treatment. Menstruation resumed and her physical and mental health started to improve. After a long 'interview' with her husband during which she learnt that he was going back to sea, she again deteriorated. It would appear from the asylum records that Maria's husband did not experience another shipwreck and that she gained strength 'working well for the bazaar' until she was able to go home for a month's trial where she 'conducted herself well' living with her father and mother as her husband had been on a voyage to Hamburg. Maria returned to the asylum and although she was still very sensitive and agitated from slight causes she was not suffering from hallucinations and was considered perfectly rational. It was decided that Maria was so well recovered that she could be discharged. It was finally noted that Maria's family were of feeble intellect and there was 'every fear that she might not be able to compete with the experiences of life successfully': 'the future however is not our province and she left the asylum today, cured.'

Victorian literature is full of references to shipwrecks because being lost at sea was a very real danger. Images of ships going aground on rocks or lost in storms were readily available in publications like *The Illustrated London News*. Novelists such as Charles Dickens and Mrs Gaskell frequently employed the motif of the shipwreck in their novels to evoke feelings of separation, loss and the danger of uncontrollable forces. In the final paragraphs of *Villette*, Charlotte Brontë writes one of the most moving narratives of lost love and it is expressed through the imagery of a supposed shipwreck. Lucy Snowe is waiting for the return of the man she loves, Paul Emmanuel. It is Autumn and by November he should have arrived home; however, the weather begins to turn foul and Lucy says, 'I know some signs of the sky; I have noted them ever since childhood. God, watch that sail! Oh Guard it!'[21] Lucy watches the sky as the storm brews:

> The wind shifts to the west. Peace, peace banshee – "keening" at every window! It will rise – it will swell – it shrieks out long: wander as I may through the house this night, I cannot lull the blast. The advancing hours make it strong: by midnight all sleepless watchers hear and fear a wild south-west storm.
>
> That storm roared frenzied for seven days. It did not cease till the Atlantic was strewn with wrecks: it did not lull till the deeps had gorged their full of sustenance. Not till the destroying angel of the tempest had achieved his perfect work, would he fold the wings whose waft was thunder – the tremor of whose plumes was storm
>
> Peace, be still! Oh! a thousand weepers, praying in agony on waiting shores, listened for that voice, but it was not uttered – not uttered till, when the hush came, some could not feel it: till, when the sun returned, his light was night to some![22]

This poetic portrayal of loss uses the language of religion in a way that would have resonated with Victorian readers. The storm is described as a destroying angel who, instead of safeguarding the faithful under his protective wings, uses them to summon up a powerful and murderous tempest. The still, gentle voice of Jesus that used the words 'peace, be still' to calm the waters in Mark 4. v.39 was drowned out until finally the storm was over and many lives had been lost. Maria Hines identified with Christ on the cross when she was in the throes of her mental disturbance brought on by her husband's shipwreck. This type of mental anguish was taken up as a motif and expressed in literature. Likewise, the fictional Lucy Snowe felt the power of the avenging angel whose force could silence even the voice of Christ as she waited for her true love to return to her.

Feelings of sin, guilt and religious despair were largely a result of the powerful influence of religion and religious education especially on women. Young, nervous females under the influence of religion were particularly susceptible.[23] The period was one of religious upheaval and gave rise to many a 'religious wave'. The nineteenth century was marked by a revival of religious activity and preachers toured the land looking for converts. Methodism, Calvinism, the Baptists and the evangelical wing of the Church of England were all on the rise and later in the century, the high church Anglo-Catholics were brought into prominence by the Oxford movement. The various denominations differed from each other in their organization and doctrine, but their moral teaching on heaven, hell, sin and redemption was fairly uniform. This activity meant that religion was constantly in the forefront of current thinking and moral instruction and must have influenced the thoughts and language of countless patients who were experiencing mental illness, causing them to be diagnosed with religious mania or excitement.

4

Evangelical Sunday School Teaching:
Lessons for Girls

Little girl, here is a book entitled the 'Child's Guide;'[1] read it with prayer,
especially that part containing 'an account of the awful and sudden death of
Martha G –,naughty child addicted to falsehood and deceit.
With these words, Mr. Brocklehurst put into my hand a thin pamphlet sewn
in a cover.

Jane Eyre p. 35.

The Gloucester Journal in 1783 reported that some of the clergy in different parts of the country were establishing Sunday schools as an attempt to bring about reform of the behaviour of working-class children on the Sabbath day and to help preserve them from idleness, immorality or ignorance. This was a clear indication of the intended role of the Sunday school in the late eighteenth century. However, by the nineteenth century, writers of the periodicals and reward books[2] used in Sunday schools widened these objectives and directed their work towards the social control of young people, girls in particular, and the saving of their immortal souls. It is evident that these texts produced a reaction in several Victorian writers of fiction, especially female authors such as Charlotte Brontë.

Through the early chapters of *Jane Eyre*, Charlotte Brontë makes her reader aware of the effect of evangelical Protestantism on the lives of poor, young girls. She based the severe and cruel character of Mr Brocklehurst, the director of Lowood School where the young Jane was a pupil, on the real-life Rev. Carus Wilson (1791–1859). When Mrs Gaskell wrote her *Life of Charlotte Brontë* in 1857, she observed:

Mr. Wilson seems to have had the unlucky gift of irritating even those to whom he meant kindly, and for whom he was making perpetual sacrifices of time and money, by never showing any respect for their independence of opinion and action. He had, too, so little knowledge of human nature as to imagine that, by constantly reminding the girls of their dependent position, and the fact that they were receiving their education from the charity of others, he could make them lowly and humble. Some of the more sensitive felt this treatment bitterly, and instead of being as grateful as they should have been for the real benefits they were obtaining, their mortified pride rose up from its fall a hundred-fold more strong. Painful impressions sink deep into the hearts of delicate and sickly children.[3]

This open criticism of Carus Wilson resulted in a furore of protest from his friends and such books as *The Vindication of Carus Wilson*, written by his son-in-law, appeared in 1857.[4] Despite these remonstrations to the contrary, works, both written and edited by Rev. Wilson, clearly demonstrated that he had a pessimistic view of children, girls in particular, which led him to advocate the breaking of their will and repression of their individual spirits in order to save their eternal souls.

Although the views of Carus Wilson were made widely known through the writing of Charlotte Brontë, it is necessary to put his ideas into context in order to ascertain whether his mode of religious teaching was prevalent at this time. During the early nineteenth century a wide range of material was written for Sunday school pupils. It was a period of English history when the evangelical Sunday schools were flourishing and the evangelistic school of thought was uppermost in the Church of England. The literature consists mainly of magazines for Sunday school children and reward books which were a vital contribution to the education of the children of the poor and went a long way in indoctrinating them with language and images which most likely influenced some of those women who would end up in lunatic asylums. It was not always clear from which denomination these books were written, but as the main objective is an analysis of the evangelical way of perceiving females (frequently from disadvantaged backgrounds), the real importance lies in the fact that these religious writings were influential.

One of the problems in looking at literature which prescribed a certain way of thinking and its effect on behaviour is how to evaluate how successful it actually was, and to examine who read or even took any notice of this material. Charlotte Brontë's father, Rev. Patrick Brontë, a committed evangelical, supported the education of the poor. He founded a Sunday school in Haworth[5] and three of his children, Charlotte, Branwell and Anne, taught there. The most significant episode in Charlotte's religious upbringing was her stay at The Clergy Daughter's School Cowan Bridge, which was run by Carus Wilson. By the time she wrote *Jane Eyre*, she had become critical of the evangelical teaching of her childhood and realized that it was a method of controlling children's behaviour, particularly young girls. Brontë's novels show how she rebelled against the kind of Calvinistic teaching propounded by Wilson and her Aunt Branwell who looked after the Brontë children following the death of their mother. She was joined in her antagonism against this philosophy by George Eliot, who rejected the teachings of evangelism even though she had gone through an earlier conversion. Eliot had become captivated with evangelicalism as a young girl under the influence of an evangelical schoolmistress. She later became disenchanted for reasons that included her disappointment with evangelical social ethics and a deeper understanding of theology. Female inmates of mental asylums would have been exposed to Sunday school literature of the early nineteenth century, and the gendered responses to their illness were a direct result of evangelical feeling.

In the nineteenth century, the aim of the evangelicals was a total reform of Church and nation. This process began in the Sunday schools:

> The teachers will be expected to seek to maintain order and regularity in their respective classes, and to bring forward the children committed to their care in the various lessons and scriptural instruction of the several classes; and particularly to endeavour to lead them into an acquaintance with the state of sin and death in which they are born, and the way of salvation by Christ; and to show them the necessity of holiness of heart and life.
>
> *Rules of the Clare Sunday School* 1840.

Evangelical Christianity appealed to the emotions. Its preachers taught the doctrine of the total depravity of man and the soul of a child was seen as a battleground for the fight between God and the Devil. Evangelicals were obsessed with the judgement that awaited them at death and their lives on earth were seen as a preparation for the afterlife. They believed that every thought or action would have to be accounted for to the Almighty. Many evangelicals wanted to work for God, to do good in the world and lead useful lives; they became noted for their philanthropic works and the sincerity with which they attempted to convert their fellow sinners in order to save them from the fires of hell. This they did by preaching and by educating poor children via the Sunday school system. Another feature for which evangelical Christians were noted was their piety and seriousness, which was often interpreted as repression, bigotry and gloom,[6] as one historian has mentioned: 'They all held strict views on manners and morals, abstained from certain pleasures and were inclined to censure those who indulged in them ... conduct became a test which proved whether one belonged to God's chosen people.'[7]

Evangelical doctrines and debates permeated the Victorian world. The evangelical movement of the Anglican Church came about in response to a religion which had become lethargic and worldly; it was emphatically Protestant in spirit. It emerged in the eighteenth century largely in order to reinvigorate Methodism that had itself began as a movement of renewal in the Church of England, but, against the wishes of its founder John Wesley, later become a separate sect. The evangelical movement had much in common with Methodism, especially the Calvinistic form of Methodism. It stressed justification by faith, the experience of personal conversion, the priority of teaching over liturgy and the absolute authority of the Bible. In asylum casebooks it was not uncommon to find young women who had been severely mentally disturbed by the preachings of a Methodist minister. However, evangelicalism was not a breakaway sect as it aimed to operate within the structure of the established church. Until the Catholic-oriented movement of the Tractarians emerged in Oxford in the mid-1830s, the evangelical party was the most dynamic in the Anglican Church and its influence persisted throughout the century. In common with the evangelicals, officials of the high church also wanted to wake up, what they considered to be a sleeping church and sought to put over their ideas with considerable fervour. Women who were considered mad often claimed to have seen, or to be, the Virgin Mary, a very prominent figure High Anglican and Catholic teaching and an important biblical character.

By 1850, 2 million working-class children were enrolled in Sunday schools.[8] Nineteenth-century evangelical ideas about children were based on the nature and potential of their minds and the condition of their souls, what later was called psychology and theology. Calvinists accepted the doctrine of original sin that held that the fall of man, the result of the disobedience of Adam and Eve in the Garden of Eden, meant that there was a tendency towards evil in all humans. They believed that original sin alienated children from God and that this alienation could only be ended by a conversion experience in which the child received God's regenerating grace. While they remained outside this so-called state of grace, children were seen as incapable of acting except from self-love and so could not be considered 'good'. Calvinists also believed that proper training in obedience and self-control was essential to minimize the outward expressions of self-love which hardened the children's souls towards God. Methodists too held the doctrine of original sin and were firm believers in a proper training in early childhood which could ease the transition to a Christian adulthood; this theological framework provided the assumptions by which evangelical Sunday school organizers operated. One of their primary tasks was to impart religious knowledge to children, the knowledge necessary for eventual conversion. Sunday school teachers were encouraged by the Rev. Carus Wilson in *The Teacher's Visitor*[9] in 1844: 'Thus, you are in a peculiar manner, fellow workers with Christ; for on you is conferred the high privilege of carrying the lambs to His bosom.' In the same volume, Wilson gave his readers a brief résumé of the changing role of the evangelical Sunday school, beginning with the founding of the first Sunday schools by Raikes in 1781–1782. After the initial idea of taking a few children off the streets of Gloucester on the Sabbath, gathering them together and offering them the rudiments of education, great changes followed:

> The thousands upon thousands who have been since, and are now taught at the Sunday School the way of salvation through Christ, justify to its influence in the origin and perfection of this plan of good ... Whatever the benevolent man who instituted schools for the instruction of poor children on the Sabbath might have intended for their establishment, God most manifestly designed that they should be the chief agency of the Church in making the young acquainted with the things that concern their eternal peace. This, their history of a half-century would seem pointedly to indicate. Now their textbook is the Bible, and a Sunday school at this day is scarcely to be found to which this precious volume is not the book of books.[10]

Evangelicalism can be used as an umbrella term to cover a wide range of doctrinal positions embraced by Anglicans, Methodists and other sects on the Protestant wing of the Christian Church. Original sin can be seen as the linchpin of the evangelical creed and this doctrine not only had a strong influence on the way children were perceived but it was also very influential in shaping society's attitude to the 'fallen woman' and her illegitimate child.[11] The 'fallen woman' was a woman who had sexual knowledge outside marriage. Whether the cause woman's 'fall' had been of her own doing or whether she had been the 'victim' of a man was irrelevant. An unmarried mother was considered a 'fallen woman' and the illegitimate child was her badge of shame. Naturally, illegitimate children absorbed that shame and grew up feeling the disgrace and guilt of their mother. Because of religious teaching on marriage, chastity and purity, illegitimate children were frequently ostracized by society along with their mothers who had broken the sexual taboos created by harsh and misogynistic dogma.

Belief in eternal punishment

Eternal punishment was continually stressed and the Sunday school literature of the time was full of references to and stories about wicked children who died in a graceless state and so went to hell. This sentiment was indoctrinated into Sunday School children, a process echoed in Charlotte Brontë's novel *Jane Eyre*. In her account of the first meeting between Jane Eyre and Mr Brocklehurst, Brontë indicates her suspicion of the real feelings behind the use of the clergyman's religious jargon and his interpretation of the scripture:

> "No sight so sad as that of a naughty child," he began, "especially a naughty little girl. Do you know where the wicked go after death?"
> "They go to hell," was my ready and orthodox answer.
> "And what is hell? Can you tell me that?"
> "A pit full of fire."
> "And should you like to fall into that pit and to be burning there for ever?"
> "No, sir."
> "What must you do to avoid it?"
> I deliberated a moment; my answer when it did come, was objectionable. "I must keep in good health, and not die."[12]

The second meeting between Jane and Mr Brocklehurst at Lowood School presents Brontë with the opportunity to illustrate the blind illogicality behind many evangelical prejudices. She shows how they were elevated, by the misapplication of theological vocabulary and certain references to the Bible, into moral condemnations.[13] However, the religion of the Sunday school went deeper than the language of the Bible or moral theology; it offered its students an assurance of salvation in an unstable world fraught with death and disease.

Belief in the Second Coming served to provide a theological perspective to this period of transition and lent the evangelicals a sense of their own importance in preparing for their idea of a future evangelical paradise. Underlying these doctrines was a firm belief in the literal truth of the Bible, at least in their particular interpretation of it. Evangelical Christians agreed that the Bible was the means whereby God revealed his purpose to man and that it contained the whole truth necessary to man's salvation.

In her article in *The Westminster Review* 1855, novelist George Eliot, in her criticism of Dr Cumming, sums up how the evangelical teacher 'manipulated' the Holy Scripture:

> We need not discuss whether Dr. Cumming's interpretation accords with the meaning of the New Testament writers: we simply point to the fact that the text becomes elastic for him when he wants freer play for his prejudices, while he makes it an adamantine barrier against the admission that mercy will ultimately triumph, – that God – i.e. Love, will be all in all.[14]

As George Eliot indicates in her criticism of the evangelical teachings of Dr Cumming, 'Dr. Cumming's theory, as we have seen, is that actions are good or evil according as they are prompted or not prompted by an exclusive reference to the "Glory of God"', it was only a small step from that assumption to the justification of the low status in life of most female Sunday School scholars and their sacred duty not to attempt to rise above their given station. Instead they were duty bound to become good servants, wives and daughters as an expression of their submission to God and the teaching he handed down through the Bible.

In recent debate on social control in nineteenth-century England,[15] Sunday schools have been seen as one medium through which the lower classes potentially could be manipulated and subdued by the middle and upper classes. Sunday schools, in the company of, 'various other schemes, were used to discipline the lower orders'.[16] Disciplinary virtues of hard work and obedience were inculcated in the working class by making them believe that their chief happiness must be found in a future life, not their present one.[17] This was the message sent out by evangelical Sunday schools, a method by which the founders of these schools could influence the social behaviour of the children of poor. What is more difficult to establish is how far this teaching met with success and whether it had the power to affect the mental health of the pupils in later life. It is probable that Sunday school teachers induced a sense of guilt in their scholars so that they could then offer them a means of assuaging it.[18] However, an emotionally charged, fundamental religion that offered people the promise of a wonderful afterlife, would have been attractive to those whose ordinary lives were unpredictable and hard. The content of the literature that was produced for the Sunday scholars provides insight into the intentions of its authors.

One genre of children's evangelical literature was the cautionary tale. To the twenty-first-century reader these stories could appear crude and even amusing, but the lessons they attempted to teach must have been worrying and influential to a child's imagination:

> It's dangerous to provoke a God
> Whose power and vengeance none can tell;
> One stroke of his almighty rod
> Can send young sinners quick to hell.
> *The Children's Friend* (1838)

The literature written specifically for the use of Sunday school scholars can be divided into three categories: the tracts and reward books given to the pupils, magazines or periodicals published by church or denominational organizations, and the textbooks used by the girls and boys during school time. The first two categories contained many cautionary tales written to inculcate the tenets of evangelical morality into the pupils.

The growth of Sunday schools was almost simultaneous with the growth of publications for children. No other institution was more instrumental in bringing the printed word to the working-class child.[19] The proliferation of titles at this time suggests that there was a wide market of children who read this type of literature. But what were they supposed to learn from their reading? The preface of *The Child's Book of the Soul* (1832) explained that it was written to be used 'in the religious instruction of the lower classes of pupils in Sunday School':

> To teach a child that he has something within him distinct from the body; unlike it, wonderfully superior to it, and which will survive it after death, and live forever:- is the simple, elementary principle of all religious instruction.[20]

He added, 'Make him [the child] feel that he is not a mere animal, that he has other and higher enjoyments than those which are sensual; that he is an intellectual, moral and accountable being, destined to an endless existence beyond the grave.'[21]

This type of religious instruction pointed clearly towards an overriding interest in the spiritual health of the child and in particular, his/her immortal soul. In the pursuit of 'saving' as many children as possible, the writers of Sunday school literature produced a great many cautionary tales about 'bad children' and exemplary stories about 'good children' in the belief that young people learnt best by example. As Clara Lucas Balfour wrote in 1817: 'Emulation is the spirit most desirable to arouse in the young. That which we are constrained to approve and admire, we are led to emulate, even where imitation may not be possible.'[22]

This method of teaching has been criticized in the debate on social control in Victorian Britain. It was seen as one of the ways in which the middle and upper classes used religion to frighten the working class into submission. Whilst it is true that the cautionary tales were frequently terrifying, there was a lot of evidence to suggest that the intention of those involved in the running of the evangelical Sunday schools was to save children from eternal damnation. The social control that resulted from scaring children also had an altruistic motive prompted by the teachers' own belief in hell and damnation. Salvation entailed a degree of submission to God and those in authority and a joyful acceptance of one's place in society. Whether the social implications of this doctrine were secondary to the religious ones or vice versa is probably of very little importance to the affect these tales had on the minds of impressionable children.

Gendered cautionary tales

Girls were particularly targeted by moral tales and this was relevant to cases of women who believed that they were unpardonable sinners. The following poem was printed in a book titled, *Hints to Girls on Dress* by A Female Teacher:

> T'is not a cause of small import
> The teacher's care demands,
> But what might fill an angel's heart,
> And filled a saviour's hands.
>
> We watch for souls! for which the Lord
> Did heavenly bliss forgo,
> For souls that must hereafter live,
> In raptures or in woe.[23]

Books like the above-mentioned *Hints to Girls on Dress* suggested that girls were in danger of losing their souls for different reasons from boys. Girls were urged to follow a prescribed pattern of behaviour in order to attain eternal life. The direction for boys' social activity was given a more flexible moral structure within which they had a certain amount of freedom to interpret what it meant to be 'good' and more scope to be 'naughty' before repentance was necessary. Girls were warned against the love of fine dress, a subject that never cropped up in boys' stories: 'This has been in all ages regarded as a female propensity and it has proved ruinous to multitudes of young females.'[24] Girls were warned against 'aping their betters' or offending their benefactors by wearing clothes that were too fine for their station. The wearing of 'decent clothes' would help them find a creditable place when they went into service. A terrible fate awaited the young woman who wasted her money on vanity. Girls who did not heed this advice were crippled by rheumatism through wearing flimsy clothes, died from broken blood vessels incurred by violent coughing, or from cholera, like Sally who 'went wrong' because of her love of dress and could be seen, 'lolling out of a window, or standing at the top of an alley scantily covered by remnants of dirty, trumpery finery'. These warnings were always justified by reference to the Bible. The vain girls were likened to Jezebel (2 Kings chap. 9 v.30) and Eve was often cited as the first example of woman's sin:

Why should our garments, made to hide
Our parent's shame, provoke our pride?
The art of dress did n'er begin
Till Eve our mother learnt to spin.
When first she put the covering on,
Her robe of innocence was gone,
And yet dear children vainly boast
In the sad marks of glory lost.[25]

The style of a girl's hair was also an important indication to the state of her soul. In *Jane Eyre*, Charlotte Brontë records a scene in which Mr Brocklehurst admonishes the girls of Lowood School for the way in which they wear their hair. Julia Severn, whose hair curled naturally, attracted the greatest obloquy. Brontë used this incident to highlight the hypocrisy of a religion that found it sinful for poor girls to wear their hair long or curled, whilst the minister's daughters sported most elaborate hairstyles. Moreover, this did indeed seem to be the opinion of Rev. Carus Wilson, the 'prototype' for Mr Brocklehurst. In *A Lily among Thorns or Short Memorial of Little Jane* (1836), the moral tale to which Wilson wrote the preface, the text enthused: 'She (Jane) cut off her plaits and ribbon, because a lady visitor said that poor girls should not dress their hair in that way, especially a sick child who should be thinking of better things.'[26]

Neglect of 'better things' seemed to preoccupy the Sunday school writers who castigated young girls who failed to address high spiritual planes and abandoned their allotted domestic chores in favour of 'frippery'. A poor girl should have been making her father's dinner, cleaning the house or attending to other 'womanly duties' rather than dressing her hair:

> I have known girls spend one hour each night and morning, in dressing their hair in all manner of fantastical forms, which was a sinful waste of time, and only disfigured them when they had done it. Besides, a great quantity of hair is injurious to the health, and renders a person very liable to receive infection. This I was told by an eminent physician.[27]

In some of these stories and instructions there was a clear effort to make girls submissive to their employers and to be content with their station in life. *The Effects of Vanity* (1799) was a story about Kitty Pertly and her friend Mary Meanwell. Kitty ended up being transported to Botany Bay where she died as a result of God's vengeance against her vanity and disrespect to her superiors. Mary, who attended Sunday school and went into service with Lady Allworth, eventually became married and had a large family. Where Kitty went particularly wrong was in her desire to 'go her own way', which resulted in her dismissal from Sunday school:

> It must be particularly hurtful to the character of girls, who seldom or never can be in a state to depend entirely upon their own will; as children they are subject to their parents, and when grown up, either as servants or wives, women should reflect that it ever be their province, and entirely their chief merit to obey.[28]

Mothers too were seen as being in danger from God's vengeance if they failed to control their daughters. This was reflected in the sad story of Janey Green in *The Children's Sunday Album* (1848):

> 'For he doth not afflict willingly, nor grieve the children of men.' *Lamentations* iii.33
>
> It is a sad sight to look at Janey Green, once the brightest and healthiest girl in the village. Through her foolish, idle, giddy ways, she has become the poor, wretched object she is now.
>
> Her mother sits sadly watching her, wishing – now vainly – she had been stricter with her child; not let her have her own way, kept her in the house at work, instead of allowing her to run out at all hours when she wished, humouring her wish to stay at home instead of going to service; bitterly she repents her weakness now. The poor thing lies there, looking wistfully at some humble cottage flowers a kindly neighbour has brought her, and her mother glances from their fresh brightness to the worn and faded face of the poor girl.
>
> She has one comfort in her sorrow – she feels that as her child's body has grown weaker, her mind has strengthened, that she is wiser than she was, and that this great affliction has brought them both nearer to God – made them understand why He has thus afflicted them; and as she sits there watching her, she prays to be forgiven for her own weak indulgence of her child, and that it may please God to raise her up again, and give her grace to serve Him better, and love him more.[29]

If girls had to learn to be obedient to a temporal as well as a spiritual master, perhaps that is why they had less freedom to express themselves. Within this strict evangelical code of behaviour, they were in more danger of losing their souls than boys and therefore needed closely defined codes of conduct. This repression of the working-class female spirit and her constant fear of hell must inevitably have had a detrimental effect on girls' and women's mental health.

Wicked girls and naughty boys

In *The Child's Companion or Sunday Scholar's Reward*[30] (1824), there were several stories concerning both good and bad girls and boys. A 'good boy', Little George, had been taught the Bible so that he would not go astray. Whilst staying with his uncle, he met Harry Wilson, an older boy who tried to persuade him to go scrumping,[31] but George would not go. Harry fell out of the apple tree and was chased by the gardener while George was given an apple for being good. The message was a clear one about the merits of being honest and not being led into sin. Good Little Betsey Saunders, on the other hand, was exemplary to other girls in her manifestation of 'womanly' domestic virtues. She was the eldest of seven children in a poor family and her mother was often unwell. Betsey looked after her brothers and sisters, she rose early, fed and dressed the children and even read to them. Goodness, for the writer of these moral tales, was clearly gendered.

Samuel, a bad boy, played in the roads and the fields on the Sabbath instead of going to church. He was reproved for his behaviour but he ignored his betters. One cold Sunday in January Samuel was playing on a frozen pond all day with his eight-year-old little brother John. Even though they had been warned that the ice was thin, John jumped on it, broke it and was drowned. Samuel fell in too but did not die. The little readers were warned: 'How dreadful the thought of being called into the eternal world, while breaking the commands of God.' Boys were depicted a being naughty in a very different way from the girls. They were Sabbath breakers, they robbed birds' nests and orchards and were punished for their misdeeds, but their sins were masculine and positive. The girls were seen as being sinful in a much more negative and almost gentle way. Mary Lawson was given a dress and a bonnet that were not at all suitable for her to wear. Her mother broke the Sabbath when she worked to make the dress fit her daughter. Mary went nutting in the unsuitable clothes. Other children laughed at her and there was a thunderstorm that resulted in her clothes being ruined. Unfortunately, Mary could not manage to run to a dry place as she was impeded by her 'unsuitable' dress and so she caught cold and died. This pattern of what was acceptable behaviour for girls and boys and the difference in their 'naughtiness' or sin is repeated over and over again in these cautionary tales.

The warnings given to girls in Sunday school literature were also frequently, overtly sexualized. Girls were seen as being particularly vulnerable to temptation and generally to the wicked world of men. In *The Happy Life* (1850) young females were offered the following advice by a well-meaning older girl:

> I am sure that when girls like us do leave their homes to go into lodgings, they must run into many temptations; if they do think they are their own mistresses, there are plenty of people who will try and get them into their power, and do them harm.[32]

Girls were warned to keep away from the company of soldiers who would give them bold, coarse manners and they were to treasure what they had learnt at the Sabbath school: 'I would beg all girls who wish to take care of their money, or health, or character, to keep quite away from all tea gardens, fairs, theatre and dances.'[33] By creating an atmosphere of fear and guilt around female behaviour, nineteenth-century authors of Christian literature subjugated the will and feelings of many young women to a 'higher' authority and, perhaps unintentionally, destroyed many a girl's self-esteem.

It has to be recognized that boys too were advised to keep away from fairs and other diversions, but for different reasons. For both genders there were temptations that would lead them from the path of Christian righteousness but girls were singled out as being in constant danger of falling into sin because they were led from the paths of modesty, respectful conduct and retirement. This is illustrated by the following passage taken from 'The Sunday Scholar's Weekly Meeting' in *The Children's Friend* (1845):

> Christian ladies! Forget not our own dear English girls ... it is a work, moreover, for which woman with her warm and tender affections, her ardent feelings and untiring love is particularly fitted ... (women need to guide) many of our own gentle sex whose days of childhood are quickly passing away and who are fast growing around us into early womanhood, then to be sent out into the dangers and temptations of the world.[34]

The insistence that females should be warm, kind and loving was yet another burden that women had to bear. If they could not identify with such womanly attributes, society, the medical profession and even the law would judge them harshly. The overriding theological premise in this phrase from *The Happy Life. A Gift for Sunday Schoolgirls* (1850) helped to explain why such writers as the Rev. W. Carus Wilson felt that he had to instil the virtue of obedience into his scholars: 'All that affects me in this world is known to God, and in His time, my sorrows will be taken away and I shall have only perfect happiness forever'. So much Sunday school literature that emerged during the late eighteenth and early nineteenth centuries emphasized the eschatological importance of religion. These ideas concerning death, judgement and the final destination of the soul would have had adverse effects on impressionable readers.

Death and the Afterlife

The Rev. W. Carus Wilson was one of the most prolific writers of highly emotional and often gruesome tales concerning the accidental deaths of wicked children. These stories aimed to scare their young readers into having proper respect for heaven and hell. Born in 1791, Wilson wrote and distributed religious tracts from the age of eight. He produced the first ever religious periodicals to appear in England, *The Friendly Visitor* (1819) and *The Children's Friend* (1824), which maintained a very large circulation for over thirty years. In 1820 he founded a school for training children and teachers in Casterton in Cumbria. This was closely followed by the establishment of the Clergy Daughters' School in 1823 and its preparatory department in 1824. Wilson was not the only evangelical writer to have strong views on the afterlife, but his magazine for children, *The Children's Friend*, contained many such stories, which were aimed at the children's feelings of guilt, damnation and salvation. These stories were clearly gendered and pointed towards a belief in the total submission of girls to a higher power and a masculine God.

Cases of accidental death would have been familiar to the nineteenth-century reader of *The Children's Friend*. The stories in the magazine showed untimely deaths of sinful children as not truly accidental but the work of a vengeful God. They worked as a moral check on the social behaviour of the

Sunday school pupils in showing the futile waste of young life. In the tale
Martha Phillips (1834), Martha who was too weak to go into service used to:

> Sing foolish songs, and read bad books aloud as they sat together, or stand at
> the door looking out into the street, and learning of other idle young women
> to waste their time in dressing smart … Her heart went after vanity and folly
> and her precious soul was neglected.

Martha was sitting by herself one evening reading a foolish tale when her cap
caught fire. She rushed outside but the wind only increased the flames. Her
head and neck were 'dreadfully burnt' and 'her senses were gone'. She lingered
for three days and then died in excruciating pain. This would appear to be a
terrible punishment for a young girl who merely enjoyed foolish books and
idle company. According to the editor of *The Children's Friend*, God would
punish a female for idleness and vanity. Martha's death in this world was seen
as preferable to her surviving to commit even greater sins thereby endangering
her immortal soul.

This theological belief was further highlighted in the story of *Little Ann*,
written for the magazine by 'A Sunday School Teacher' (1833) as an example
to little girls:

> My dear children, I wish to tell you all about what the great God did in this
> village, a short time since, to a little girl, as I am hoping that it may be the
> means of hindering you from doing as she did and suffering from it.

Ann's mother had to leave home for the day. She left the children's dinner and
the house key with a neighbour. Ann, usually a good girl, was to look after
her two younger siblings. She managed to leave school early by lying that she
had to get home to light the fire and fry some potatoes. She took the key and a
candle and went into her house to light the fire. All the time God was watching!
God was worried that if Ann continued to lie, her soul would be 'cast into the
dreadful pit of fire and brimstone, prepared for liars.' So, 'in love to her poor
little soul, he caused the candle to catch her clothes on fire.' Ann was alone with
God; he did not let her die but sent a neighbour to assist her. With the help of
a man carrying water from the well they managed to put the fire out. God was
facilitating the rescue because, 'he was not willing to burn poor little Ann to
death, though he saw it was needful to burn most of her clothes off, and her

little legs and arms were sadly burnt'. Every time Ann saw her scars she would be reminded not to speak falsely. This story purported to teach children not to tell lies, but Ann's real fault was her acting on her own initiative. She was even attempting to perform a kindly act. By justifying the actions of a cruel Old Testament God, this evangelical writer imposed on the young reader his particular view of sin and punishment and its relation to the passive role of girls in society.

In 'Hints on Sunday Schools', a section of *The Children's Friend* (1838), informed the reader, 'Our lads may yet seem rude and boisterous, and yet without any serious hearty feelings towards God. And our girls may be vain and giggly.' These 'rude and boisterous' boys were portrayed in stories like *Boy and Fireworks* in which H.L. was badly burnt by fireworks igniting in his pocket when he attempted to hide them from his mother. He did not die but had to stay in bed for a year. H.L. suffered in his body, but the reader is invited to consider that it would have been much worse if he had gone to hell. That lesson was repeated in a short address, within a sermon, to two boys confined in the stocks for stealing apples on the Sabbath: 'If you die in your sins, you will be confined in the prison of Hell through the dark night; not for a few hours only, as at present, but for never ending eternity.' In *The Sabbath Profanator* (1837), boys were drowned when swimming on the Sabbath and others died in a house fire whilst in a state of sin; however, the worst story relating to boys was the *Tale of Daniel Rutherford*. Daniel's sin lay not in his wish to improve himself but in the fact that he had rejected his religion and had attempted to rise above his allotted station in life. According to the story, the rot set in early in his life when Daniel failed to attend Sunday school in order to go and rob birds' nests on the Sabbath. Daniel was twelve years old when he first started Sunday school; indeed, the editor gave personal details so that he was positively identified. Initially he was a good boy and a diligent pupil. However, he became 'careless', immune to punishment and laughed at any attempts to discipline him. Daniel lied about the real reason he was absent from school and both his father and the Sunday school superintendent chastised him to no avail. He left the school to become a carpenter and moved to the village where he met and befriended a medical student and decided to become a doctor too, even though his father was poor. For two years he worked as a carpenter during the day and studied Latin at night. The writer commented, 'Alas! If he had used the same diligence in his proper station, the same fervour in seeking the Lord, he would have been the happiest of men.' Daniel's Latin books kept him from church and he was influenced by Tom Paine, 'the infidel', and his followers who flattered him. Eventually, on a lone heath in a clearing in Etterick Forest he lit a fire and burnt a Bible. After this terrible deed, Daniel went from bad to worse. He received a legacy from a relative, which enabled him to go to medical school in Edinburgh where, during his first year he progressed in his studies but 'also in sin'. By the second year his health and his money were gone; he was diseased and in debt. His one remaining friend recorded Daniel's dying words:

> The terrors of death have fallen upon me – he taketh me away as with a whirlwind, in his wrath. He maketh my loins to shake … O! that I had never, never, never been born. O! that I had never left Sunday school.

Daniel died a horrible death, and afterwards, we were told that, 'the spirit of Daniel had fled!' Daniel was an active, defiant, positive boy, who lived life to the full, yet his sins led him to hell. His fault lay in failing to recognize his place in life and attempting to climb above his station.

Infant mortality was very high amongst the families of the working-class poor in the early and mid-nineteenth century. In Manchester in 1840, fifty-seven out of a hundred working-class children died before they were five years old. It is not surprising therefore to find that the Victorians had what almost amounted to an obsession with death. The deathbed scene became a familiar convention in the imaginative literature of the time, in both secular and evangelical narrative. Children played a particular part in this 'cult of the dead' and the hope of family reunion in heaven was frequently expressed in both secular and religious writing. That children would remain in their childish form in the afterlife was a prevalent belief, those who had died young would wait in heaven to welcome their parents. This hope was reflected in the popular Sunday school hymn, 'There's a Friend for Little Children'[35]:

> There's a home for little children
> Above the bright blue sky,
> Where Jesus reigns in glory,
> A home of peace and joy;
> No home on earth is like it, nor can with it compare;

For everyone is happy, nor could be happier there.
(*Hymns Ancient and Modern*)

For the evangelicals, heaven was the reward of the blessed. The afterlife was seen as a transcendent, spiritual dimension rather than a mere projection of earthly desires. As death was the necessary consequence of original sin, it took on a deep significance. On his or her deathbed, the child was perceived as very close to the final judgement that would determine whether their ultimate destination was to be 'above the bright blue sky' or eternal torment. The importance of a pious death to evangelicals, particularly the Rev. Carus Wilson, motivated them to evolve a ritual that would help dying children and their families cope with such a familiar and heart-rending situation. Whilst it is possible these stories were written in simple language that would have been used by children themselves, it is difficult to believe that this pietistic style was typical of the way that dying children spoke and behaved.[36] It is more likely that the religion of the Sunday school in its eschatological form provided a way of dealing with the fear of death, and the involvement of the community of the school helped their dying pupils in their last moments. A typical example of this style can be seen in a story written by Carus Wilson about the death of a little girl: One morning she said to her mother, 'I am very happy; for tonight, I have been thinking and dreaming all about heaven and about the angels, and soon I shall be one there.'[37]

The only really detailed description of the afterlife in the New Testament is found in The Book of Revelation chapter seven which is referred to by the Victorian writer Mrs Gaskell in her novel *North and South*:

> But where would I hear such grand words of promise -hear tell o'anything so far different fro' this dreary world, and this town above a', as in Revelations? Many's the time i've repeated the verses in the seventh chapter to myself, just for the sound. It's as good as an organ, and as different from everyday, too No, I cannot give up Revelations. It gives me more comfort than any other book i' the Bible.[38]

Mrs Gaskell was a Unitarian who did not believe in hell and the last judgement yet she chose to put these words into the mouth of the dying Betsy Higgins because she understood the teaching offered by the evangelicals to the working-class poor. Nineteenth-century evangelical Christians believed firmly in a future life consisting of both a heaven and a hell. They based their belief on the Bible but seemed to overlook the interpretation of The New Testament, particularly in the deciphering of Jesus's teaching about 'The Kingdom' in his parables and veiled references to the afterlife. A shared vocabulary, which was characteristically Victorian, provided writers with a cluster of key ideas and symbols associated with death and the future life.[39] The words of the dying held special significance in the nineteenth century and writers of Sunday school literature helped reinforce their importance.

The last words uttered by Helen Burns in *Jane Eyre* could have been lifted from the pages of *The Children's Friend* apart from the fact that there is no mention of hell. Charlotte Brontë, like her friend Mrs Gaskell, rejected the idea of hell and believed that every human soul would ultimately be reconciled to God through the love and mercy of Jesus. She believed that if a person died in a sinful state, they would be corrected by God, but no punishment would last forever or result in the destruction of the soul, which is immortal. Brontë uses the voice of Helen Burns to put forward her idea of universalism and her rejection of the evangelical notion of eternal retribution:

> But where are you going to Helen? Can you see? Do you know?
> I believe, I have faith: I am going to God.
> Where is God? What is God?
> My maker and yours; who will never destroy what he has created. I rely implicitly on his power, and confide wholly in his goodness: I count the hours till that eventful one arrives which shall restore me to him, reveal him to me.
> You are sure, the Helen, that there is such a place as heaven; and that our souls can get to it when we die?
> I am sure there is a future state; ...[40]

In this scene Helen is happy to die because she believes that she is going to God. This 'happiness' was part of the formula of children's deathbed stories.

Usually there was a type of catechism by a minister or pious friend, which was addressed to the dying child. A real deathbed dialogue, which took place between the Rev. Carus Wilson and a young pupil from the Clergy School at Cowan Bridge, was recorded in *The Children's Friend* by Wilson himself. It shows the ritual questioning and the expected answers of a dying child:

Sarah, are you happy?

Yes, very happy sir.

And what is it that makes you so happy?

Because Jesus Christ died to save me, and he will take me to heaven.

And will he save all men?

No, sir, only those who trust in him.

And do you trust in him?

I hope I do, sir.[41]

Sarah died suffering greatly from inflammation in the bowels. Her teachers said that she was an exemplary child. She was dutiful, industrious and never gave her superiors any trouble. She even told her schoolfellows to humble their pride. It was hardly surprising that Rev. Carus Wilson wrote of her: 'I bless God, that he has taken from us the child of whose salvation we have the best hope; and may her death be the means of rousing many of her school fellows to seek the Lord while he may be found.' It may seem surprising to read thanks for the death of a child. However, for Wilson, who was secure in the knowledge that Sarah would be in heaven because in life she had demonstrated all the Christian qualities that would ensure her entry, it would have been something to rejoice over. Her life and more importantly her death served as a good example to other girls in her position.

In *Women Worth Emulating* (1877), Clara Lucas Balfour, a prolific writer of literature with a Christian message, urged girls to follow the example of the hymn writer Miss Charlotte Elliott (1789–1871). They were told that: 'It was her sense of sin that developed in her mind, those lovely, yearning, submissive thoughts which are expressed in her beautiful hymns.' These 'submissive thoughts' were perceived as being particularly appropriate to females. The following sentence from the same book further supports the argument that the instruction found in Sunday school literature was heavily gendered: 'It is a sad fact that inherited maladies or constitutional defects do fall to the lot of very many of the female sex.' The common phrase, which has passed into a motto 'The Suffering Sex', may have been intended to apply to the sympathetic mind of a woman quite as much as to the body. Sickness was seen as good for women; solitude, suffering and self-communion matured a fine mind and sublimated a sweet spirit – in the sick chamber, a woman dwelt with God. It was also the lot of the woman to inherit the female maladies of the reproductive organs be they physical or psychological.

The interest in pious deaths and suffering can be seen as an attempt to evolve a ritual form of dying to help families cope with the fact that so many children died young. There was a strong emphasis on fatalism and the acceptance of one's lot as the will of God. Therefore, the child should be happy to participate in the spiritual process of suffering and death and to identify with Christ on the cross. Because death was seen as the necessary punishment for original sin, it was important that even the youngest child should try to avoid being in a state of sin, just in case he or she should die suddenly and be called to judgement. Boys were far more positively good, generous, honest and supportive to their families, whereas girls' goodness lay in humility, submissiveness and avoidance of frivolous behaviour. In cautionary tales, sin and goodness were, therefore, definitely gendered states.

The good wife, daughter and female servant

The good wife and the good daughter were common tropes in the religious literature of the time. Women were seen as a means by which men could come to God. 'The Good Daughter', a story from *The Children's Sunday Album* (1848),[42] tells the story of Margaret Holt who was the daughter of 'one of the worst characters in the village' and how she brought about her father's salvation. The parson had tried to rescue the man's soul, but in vain; he could only succeed in persuading him to send his little girl to school. There the child first heard of God and how he 'came to save us all'. When Margaret came home from school she thought that she would try and teach her father what she had learnt. At first he refused to listen and laughed at his daughter, but Margaret persevered and at last had the pleasure of seeing him go to church and persuading him to listen whilst she read out loud to him the Bible stories which were so important to her. Margaret's words and entreaties had more power over her father than anything else. When he was quite an old man and Margaret a happy wife and mother, he used to go down to her cottage and feel wiser and better for seeing her sitting at the open window, work in hand, 'her soft bright eyes every moment resting on the open bible from which, she said, she always got a lesson, a warning, or a blessing for every moment of her life'.

The teaching of this Sunday school literature and the prescriptions of the evangelical writers influenced the children who read them, infusing them with feelings of sin and guilt which would have lasting effects on women in later life. The work of the Rev. W. Carus Wilson seems to have been a fairly typical (if at times a little extreme) example of the evangelical teaching of the nineteenth century. His obituary in *The Christian Observer* March 1860 mentions that he was originally rejected for Anglican ordination because of his 'Calvinistic opinions'. The obituarist remarked, 'The principles of evangelical truth [according to Carus Wilson] were far more singular, even thirty years ago, than happily they have become since,' an assumption that although Wilson was inclined to severity, his teaching, nevertheless, embodied the principles of evangelical truth. Even as recently as 1960 Wilson's teaching has been justified as being genuine in its religious intention. He was praised for caring for the worldly needs of his charges, as well as being anxious to 'save their souls from the fires of hell and to secure for them eternal life'. In *Jane Eyre*, Charlotte Brontë does not exaggerate Wilson's teaching on damnation to all sinners, nor his earnest entreaties to the girls to repent before it was too late. Carus Wilson sometimes found it necessary to expel girls who showed no sign of improving their evil dispositions that made them dangerous companions.[43]

Wilson's attitude reflected the common contemporary idea that children, particularly girls, were expected to be virtuous and that those who were not, were punished in this life and would receive penalties of severe torment in the life to come. Charlotte Brontë's portrayal of Carus Wilson in the guise of Mr Brocklehurst in *Jane Eyre* is faithful to his character. His religious fanaticism and his belief in the intrinsic sinfulness of children were directed towards poor, working-class girls and consequently affected how he thought they should behave in order to attain eternal life.

Girls who were entering households as domestic servants were thought to be in particular need of the beneficial advice of Sunday school teaching. In *The Young Servant's Friendly Instructor* (1835), which was recommended in a Sunday school magazine, 'Aunt Susan' gave advice to 'Jane' who was being sent into service. The 'aunt' emphasized that she was not training her niece to become a lady:

Then what with the Sunday school and what with a little teaching on week evenings, they pick up learning enough to fit them to fill their own station in life, I am sure I have no wish to set them above it. Then there is one most important thing that should never be lost sight of. The greatest happiness of this life consists in an advancing preparation for, and looking forward to, a better.[44]

By offering the prospect of a better life in the future, the religious teacher could attempt to persuade the girls to become submissive in this one:

Obedience to employers – not to obey is a transgression of the commandment of God our saviour … Christian servants are bound to obey the doctrines of God their saviour in all things. It is both pleasing and profitable to trace the precepts for their various duties in the sacred scriptures.[45]

To substantiate her instruction, 'Aunt Susan' took the Bible and she and 'Jane' made a little table of references to passages which contained special direction or encouragement to servants. At the end of their studies 'Jane' is exhorted to respect what she has learnt:

In a word, do everything in view of that great account which you must one day render, when masters and servants shall stand before the bar of God, and be judged according to the deeds done in the body, whether they be good or whether they be evil.[46]

Children were encouraged to be 'good' by the writers of evangelical Sunday school literature for fear for their immortal souls. Religion was used to frighten them into accepting their station in life and to behave accordingly. Rigid doctrines of evangelical Christianity lent authority to the teachings of men such as Rev. Carus Wilson. These doctrines gave substance to the view that working-class girls should be submissive and not try to ape their social betters. They were bound by the God's will to be deferent to their superiors and modest in their dress. Working-class boys, however, were portrayed as active, positive and assertive. Their negative attributes were seen only when they put themselves in danger, thieved or rejected religion.

Frightening children with warnings of hell was common practice amongst evangelical Protestants during the nineteenth century and it has been argued that hellfire preaching, the similar Sunday School cautionary tales and deathbed calls to repentance were not necessarily effective in the fight against sin.[47] On the other hand, because heaven and hell are intangible and invisible concepts, they could become terrifyingly real in the fertile imagination of a young person. Charlotte Brontë was not working class but it appears from her writing that the evangelical influence she underwent as a child had a lasting influence on her. Such fears acted as a control on behaviour and formed the basis of a language they could be employed to express emotions that were not fully understood. It was hardly surprising, therefore, that the language of religion was used to voice the overwhelming and frightening feelings of those who were suffering from mental health problems. The profound sense of sin and guilt was articulated mainly by women, whereas men vocalized through religion in a more dynamic and judgemental way.

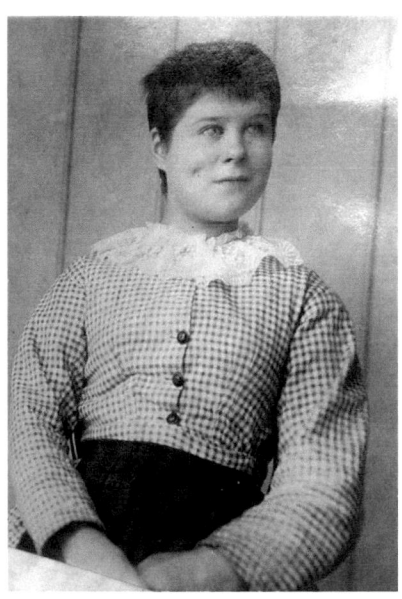

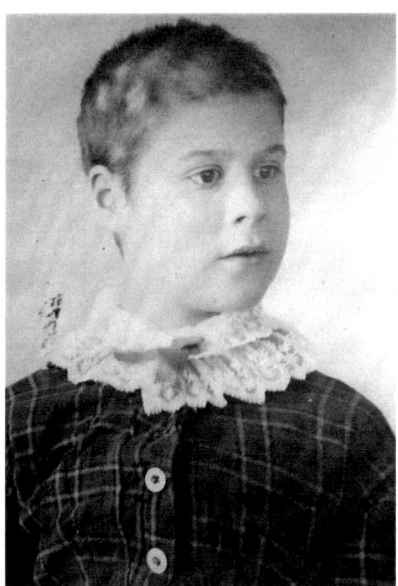

Plates 1 and 2 An example of head shaving.

Charlotte Rowe was a fourteen-year-old, single, domestic servant who lived in the Marylebone workhouse. She was diagnosed with sub-acute melancholia and had been caught attempting to throw herself out of the window.

Whilst in the asylum, she improved. She ate well and was usefully employed. After three months she was discharged, considered recovered.

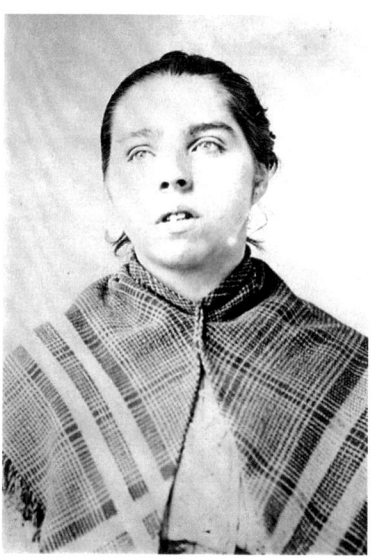

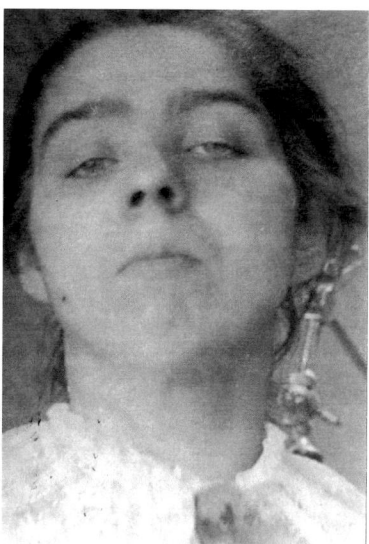

Plates 3 and 4 Example of the use of a head brace, shown in the second photograph.

Ellen Constable was a seventeen-year-old single, illegitimate servant. She said that she was in the Lord Jesus Christ's house and had other religious delusions.

Her mother, Harriet Bryant, said that Ellen wandered away from home and was absent all night. In the morning the police sent a telegram stating that her daughter had been detained as a lunatic.

After one year in the asylum, Ellen was discharged, considered recovered.

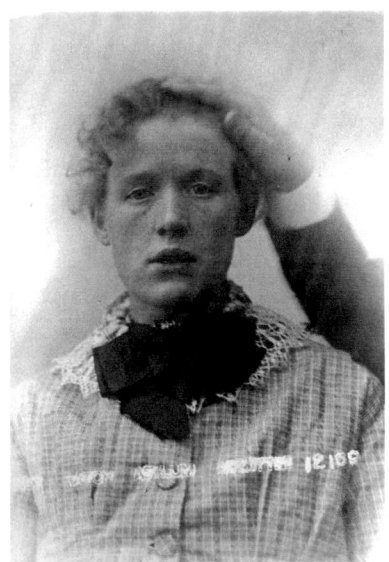

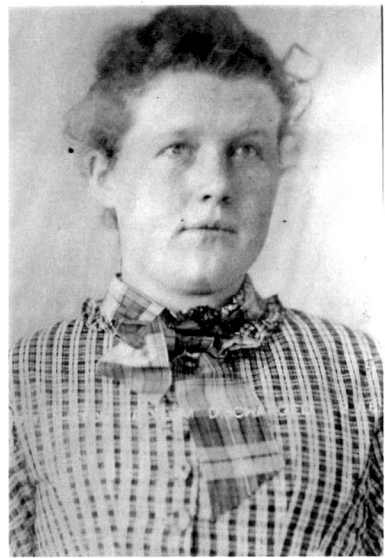

Plates 5 and 6 Ellen Roche was a single, Roman Catholic servant aged nineteen who lived in the St. Giles workhouse. Her mother was confined in the Cork County Lunatic Asylum. She was very 'excitable, noisy, loquacious and incoherent' and frequently burst into tears. She had the delusion that she had 'killed thousands'. When the doctors asked her how she had done this, she said, 'I became a woman in 1899. I have killed doctors. Send for the priest.' (In 1899 she would have been fourteen years old).

Ellen's employer said that she had to be restrained as she had threatened to cut her own throat.

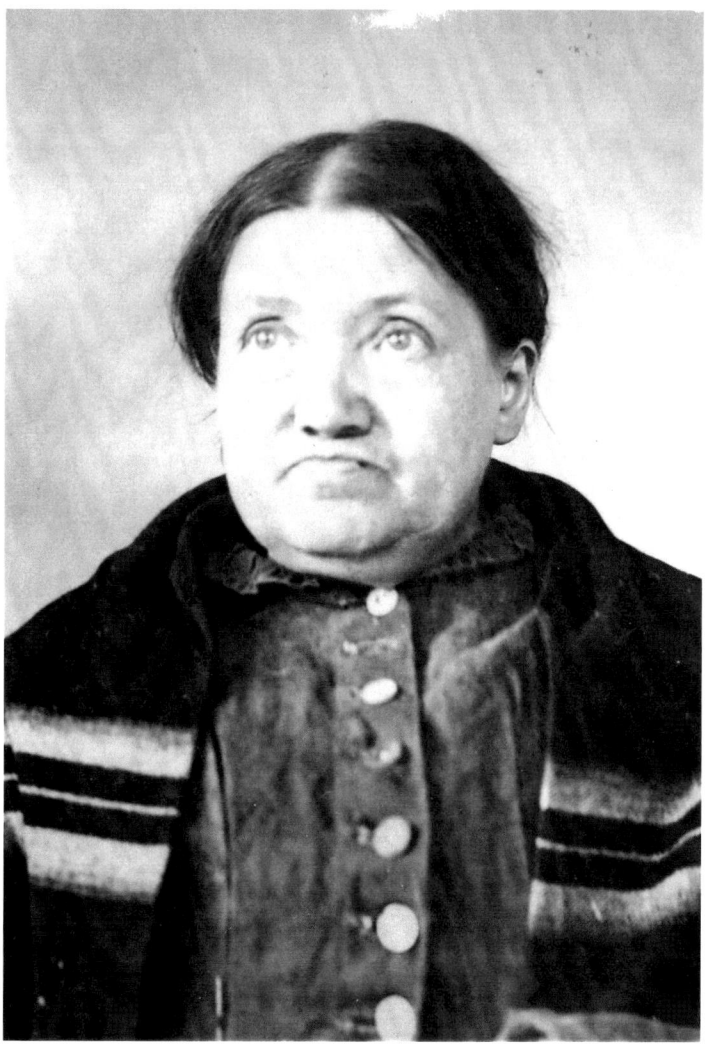

Plate 7 Ellen Wright was a sixty-four-year-old single cook who had no known relatives. She was under the delusion that she had something stuck inside her vagina and the only way to dislodge it was to have sexual intercourse with a man. She was said to have enticed men with drink to persuade them to have sexual intercourse with her in the open street and stated that she heard voices urging her to do this.

Her landlady, Catherine Russell, affirmed that Ellen was continually bringing men in to the house for immoral purposes saying that it was to cure her complaint. Mrs. Russell also said that Ellen heard voices singing to her, upbraiding her for not getting a husband. Mrs. Warren, a married woman living in the same house, said that Ellen had asked for the loan of her husband and her eldest son to 'build her up from below' by having sex with her. She was reported to have solicited, in a manner described as insane, every strange man she met.

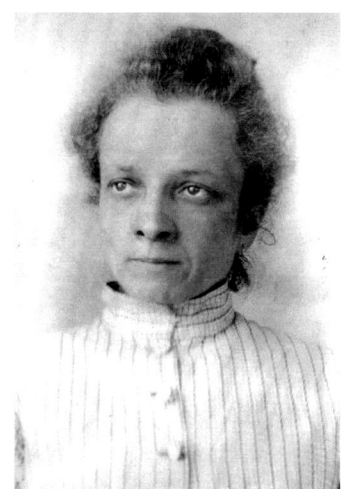

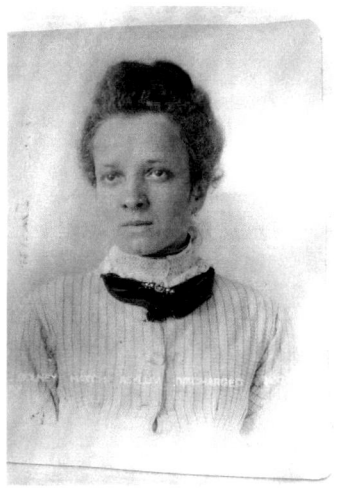

Plates 8 and 9 Fanny Smith was a single servant aged thirty-eight who was diagnosed as suffering from religious mania. She said she commenced to hear voices that told her to kneel down and pray, five months prior to her admittance to the asylum. She described the voices as being like 'scripture voices' and she believed that they had started because she had troubled her mother by screaming. She had delusions about the end of the world and other troubling subjects.

Fanny described her mental state as retribution from God, 'I feel I am going under some punishment, for some woman said I was a heretic. I think she had a bad influence over me'. She heard voices calling in the street that the Messiah had come and she insisted that she had seen a number of people burning up in flames. Her sister and mother said that she had been asking strange religious questions.

Fanny spent two months in Colney Hatch before being discharged deemed recovered.

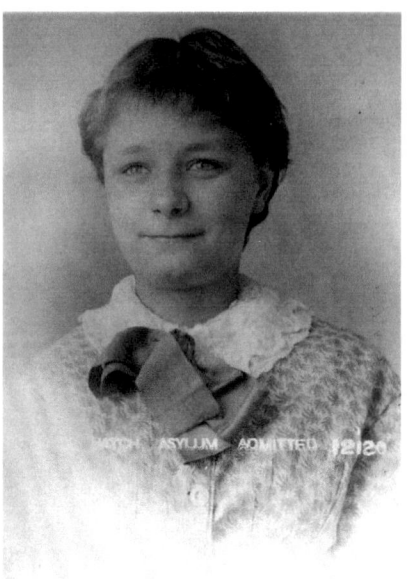

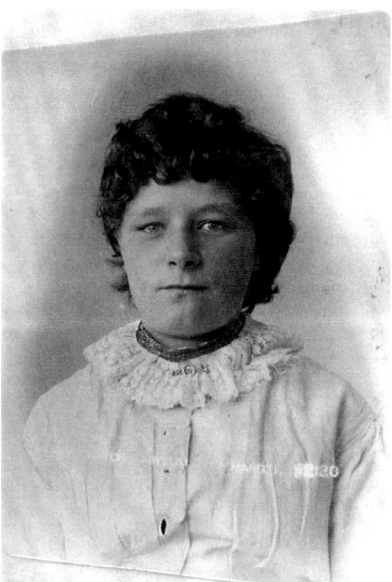

Plates 10 and 11 Florence Fuggles was a single servant aged fourteen. She said that her parents and her siblings came to her bedside to keep her awake by talking to her. She saw 'queer figures' on the walls and ceiling and her ideas on time and place were very confused. She refused to eat her dinner because the parrot told her not to do so.

Florence was kept in the asylum for three months. She worked in the laundry and became 'bright, cheerful and coherent'. She was discharged regarded cured.

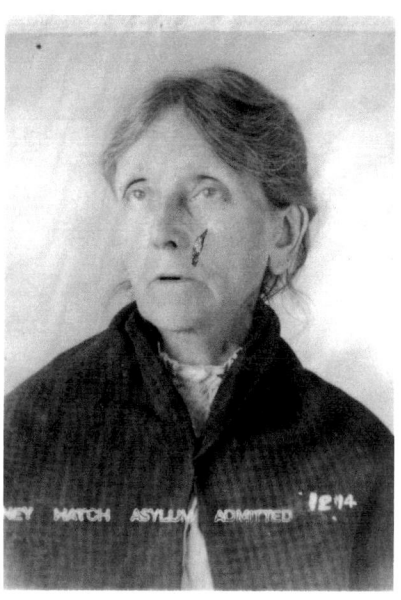

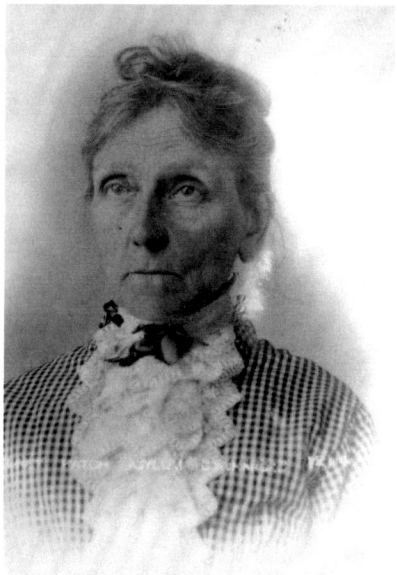

Plates 12 and 13 Example of an elderly, spinster governess.

Francis Elizabeth Burton was a sixty-year-old, single governess who was diagnosed with religious mania. She was walking along Church Park in Stoke Newington, London, when she heard the devil whispering to her, urging her to commit suicide. She imagined that people were staring at her as she walked along the street. She was under the delusion that a woman was plotting to chloroform her.

After three months in the asylum, Francis was discharged, considered recovered.

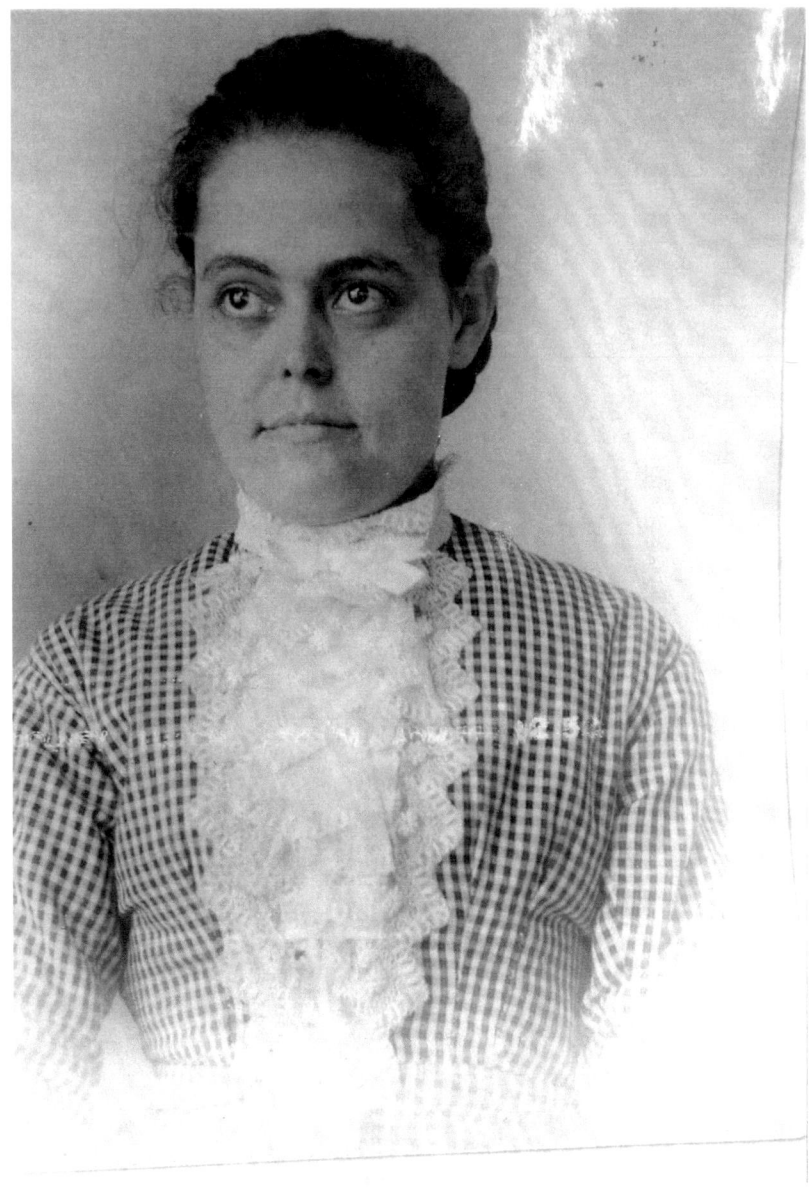

Plate 14 Example of a young, uneducated woman knowing her Bible and using its language to express her distress.

Henrietta Taylor was a twenty-three-year-old single, servant. She said that she could hear God speaking to her and she imagined she was Elijah and that she was going to Heaven in a chariot. Most of the time she was said to be 'quiet mentally' and she ate and slept well. However, she remained in the asylum for nine years when, aged thirty-two, she died in the Colney Hatch fire of 1903.

Physical Illness

There is a something which I dread
It is a dark, a fearful thing;
It steals along with withering tread,
Or sweeps on wild destruction's wing.

That thought comes o'er me in the house
Of grief, of sickness, or of sadness;
'T'is not the dread of death – t'is more,
It is the dread of madness

Poem by Lucretia Maria Davidson 1825.
Written when dying from tuberculosis.[1]

Physical causes of mental illness were well documented in the nineteenth century and most of them were specifically relevant to women because of their reproductive system and perceived frailty. As Jane Ussher noted in her book *The Psychology of the Female Body*: 'All women's madness, illness and deviant behaviour was traditionally located in the womb; malfunctions or diseases of the reproductive organs were seen as being at the root of women's "deviances". Conversely, the reproductive capability was seen as being detrimentally affected by women's deviant behaviour.'[2]

Whilst this belief about women's reproductive systems was reflected in the asylum case notes there were other, sometimes unusual, physical reasons given for women's madness. One of the most common of these symptoms was that of 'costiveness' or, to give it its modern term, constipation. According to Edward Jukes, surgeon and inventor of the stomach pump:

Costiveness may be considered, from whatever cause it arises, to be the forerunner and the foundation of most disorders that render our lives wretched, or terminate fatally. ... Females in particular should be careful to attend to those causes, which are liable to derange their digestive organs, as they have much more to encounter with, as affects their general health, than the other sex, and less constitutional power to resist the havoc of disease. ... Females in this country are more subject to constipation than males, owing both to constitutional weakness and to their employments being of a more sedentary description and seldom connected with active bodily exertion. The effect also of constipation is more injurious to females, owing to the various constitutional changes to which they are subject, particularly at the menstrual periods and during pregnancy.[3]

As William Hewitt (1865) put it: 'That he would have a clear head must have a clean stomach.' To this he added, 'He will not have a clean stomach without he has clean bowels.'[4]

With such theories around insanity being in vogue at the time, it is surely unsurprising that when women presented with inexplicable pain they were frequently treated for hysteria or hypochondria and were purged by the employment of enemas or laxatives, bled, or in extreme cases underwent a clitoridectomy.[5] In setting out his treatment of hysterical girls, George Savage, superintendent of Bethlem wrote:

Food, warmth, exercise and absence of friends are the first essentials, and next the ovarian or uterine trouble must be attended to ... If it be found that there is tenderness about the ovaries, a blister or leeches may be applied in the inguinal regions and the patient kept in bed for a short time.[6]

Savage was talking about girls who were neurotic or had an 'hysterical history'; he added that the symptoms that they might present with 'may develop, either from religious motives or from some feeling of gastric uneasiness'. His prescription for warmth and rest may have been beneficial to those women who had a bodily illness, but his other 'cures' would have been harsh and, in all probability, detrimental.

The danger of treating certain bodily symptoms as indications of madness was manifested in the case notes of women who died from a physical illness, particularly cancer and pulmonary disease. Some of the very quick cures recorded in asylum case notes appear, at first sight, to be the result of the patient being treated for physical ill health or fatigue. Luckily for the patient, when these treatments were successful she was relieved of mental distress as well. The misdiagnosis of their principal illness meant that many women, who were perceived to be hysterical, were erroneously admitted to lunatic asylums. One such speedy recovery was that of Rosa Lusner, an eighteen-year-old Jewish sempstress, said to be suicidal and dangerous, who became a patient of Bethlem in August 1858. The doctor's certificate stated that Rosa was excitable and 'wandering in her manner'. She said that the three persons in the room with her were respectively the Devil, God Almighty and Jesus Christ, which was surprising as she was a Jew and would not have recognized Jesus as the Messiah. Even though Rosa's notes were very scanty, we learn that she attempted to throw herself out of the window, cut her own throat, was 'troubled by religion', was dirty, noisy at night and that all this led to a state of rigidity. What precipitated Rosa's trouble or what caused her to stop menstruating and to be so distressed that she suffered from catalepsy was not mentioned. Her health improved in the asylum and it was noted that 'her bowels were cleared and catamenia returned'. By December 1858 Rosa was discharged 'cured'.

One nineteenth-century theory was that these physical conditions, cessation of the menses and muscular rigidity, were linked to hysteria brought on by shock, depression, or the repression of sexual feeling.[7] Robert Brudnell Carter's[8] book, *On the Pathology and Treatment of Hysteria*, was based on his experiences in clinical practice and he defined hysteria as:

> A disease which commences with a convulsive paroxysm ... This paroxysm is witnessed under various aspects, and in various degrees of severity, being limited, in some cases, to a short attack of laughter or sobbing; and in others, producing very energetic involuntary movements, maintained during a considerable time, and occasionally terminating in a period of catalepsy or coma.[9]

Brudnell Carter also described the workings of emotion and said that 'the natural tendency of an emotion is to discharge itself either through the muscular, the secreting, or the sanguiferous system', a theory that would explain both the rigidity of Rosa Lusner's muscles and the resumption of her periods.

Religious monomania had been considered a realistic diagnosis in certain types of symptoms, although often physicians failed to connect mental illness to physical symptoms in a patient. The term 'monomania' was first employed by the French psychiatrist Jean-Étienne Esquirol (1770–1840) during the early nineteenth century and became a fashionable diagnosis. It was also known as partial insanity because it was supposed to affect only part of the brain leaving the patient rational in other matters.[10] It became a useful identification for mind doctors when they were presented with patients who showed a tendency to obsess about a particular subject and physicians had come to use the term as applicable, mainly to women, who showed any signs of preoccupation with religion, as in the case of Mary Wills, a sixty-year-old married staymaker who was identified as suffering from religious monomania and 'restlessness' when she was put into Bethlem in January 1856. According to the second certificate from Dr Strange, Mary believed, as so many other female patients, that she had committed some great sin against God which could not be forgiven and so her soul was lost. She also believed that people were employed to cut her throat. However, Mary's case notes seemed to contradict the certification of madness. They stated that she was an elderly invalid with severe bronchitis and other physical problems. She had to be warmed up before they could begin treating her, which suggested that she was suffering from hypothermia on admittance. The Bethlem medical staff, contrary to the evidence of the committing doctors, could find no signs of insanity and believed that she had been placed in the asylum because she was a problem to look after, an inconvenience. What Mary needed was to be cared for as an invalid. She was desperate to stay in Bethlem and cried a lot when she knew that she was going to be discharged, whilst she was 'uncured' in January 1857 exactly a year after her admittance.[11] We do not know where Mary went or whether she lived or died. In this case, the asylum realized that the patient was not mentally ill yet cared for her for twelve months. It can only be surmised that the doctors who signed her original certificates of insanity colluded with the family to have Mary shut away as a religious monomaniac.

Instead of looking to see if there was a physical illness to be addressed before committing a woman to an asylum, doctors often seemed to either take the word of the afflicted person's relatives or see her religious ramblings as a sure sign of insanity. A similar case of apparent misdiagnosis of a physically ill woman was that of 44-year-old married hawker of twine, Susannah Downing, who came from Ipswich. She had seven children, the youngest of which was just four years old. She was said to have had a previous attack of mental illness eight years earlier, which resulted in her being confined to Bethlem for one year. No indication was given in her notes as to the causes of the attack. With seven children, the last one having been born when she was forty, Susannah was, in all likelihood, suffering with serious, physical exhaustion. By the time she arrived back in Bethlem in February 1857, she was in poor bodily health, suffering from anxiety, considered dangerous to others but not suicidal. Her first certificate, signed by Dr Webster Adams from St. Clements County Asylum in Ipswich, stated that Susannah's mind was disturbed on 'religious subjects and her conduct was violent'. She believed that members of her family were 'angels and devils'. Similar symptoms had been displayed in her previous confinement. Her second certificate signed by William Elliston of Ipswich mentioned that Susannah had been in Union House, the Ipswich workhouse at that time. She had been 'most outrageous', biting and striking at all within her reach, talking incoherently on religion and 'conversing with angels'. However, the staff caring for her also recorded that Susannah was in a bad state of health, untidy and sometimes dirty due to her physically frail state. She was also under-nourished and would not eat much whilst under their care. As she grew weaker, she stopped taking food, only drinking very small quantities of beef tea and wine. She took to her bed and after nine days, on 18 February 1857, she died of apparent exhaustion and malnutrition; the cause of death was given as pneumonia and acute melancholia. It was not clear whether she stopped eating because she was severely depressed, because she was suffering from pneumonia or if her poor bodily health was the reason for her melancholy. However, whether or not she was suffering from mental illness, there is no doubt that she would have been much better served by a general hospital where she would have been treated for her physical illness before being assessed for possible confinement in an asylum for the insane.

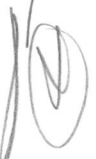

Cork lunatics

Roman Catholic patients in the Cork District Lunatic Asylum in Ireland expressed their mental and physical health problems in a different language from their mainly Protestant, corresponding patients in English asylums. Sometimes they would speak about the Pope but were more likely to reference local folk law or even the Queen of England when they were attempting to express their feelings and pain. However, like their English counterparts, some of them were also confined in a mental institution when they were suffering from distressing physical ailments which were perceived as indications of madness. At least two cases emerge of women being admitted to a lunatic hospital when they were, in fact, suffering from the painful end symptoms of cancer. In 1894 a 36-year-old female, 'Annie',[12] entered the Cork Asylum suffering from syncope (fainting), irregular heart action and a feeble pulse. No explanation was given as to why she was sent to the asylum and not treated in a general hospital, nor was any reference made to her mental condition. The treatment given to Annie was to warm her feet and a whiskey and mustard plaster applied to her cardiac region. Whiskey was frequently used as a cardiac stimulant in the nineteenth century as it was believed to increase the heart rate. The first indication of any madness was when her notes stated that Annie appeared to be rambling. She said that men were 'making game of her'. Her bodily health began to improve but relapsed as she started repeatedly vomiting, whereupon she was transferred to hospital where she continued to vomit.[13] By November 1896, Annie's health had deteriorated and the asylum contacted her relatives, the priest was called, and she received the anointing of the sick, an indication that she was believed to be seriously ill and possibly near to death. It was noted that she was still 'looking thin and that her mental condition had not improved'. Again, there was no description of Annie's so-called mental condition; we only learnt that her wheezing and vomiting attacks disappeared under proper treatment, although the treatment was not specified. As she became weaker with severe pains in her abdomen, she was given an injection of morphine and a linseed poultice was applied to her stomach. In March 1898 she again received the anointing of the sick and her friends were informed of the seriousness of her condition. Six days later, Annie rallied, but recovery was brief, and in September 1898 she died from 'chronic brain deterioration and carcinoma of the stomach'. What had the doctors meant by 'brain deterioration'? Did Annie have a neurodegenerative disease or even a brain tumour? The only reference to her mental health was soon after her admittance when she said that men were making 'a game of her', which could, of course, be a reference to real abuse in the ward. However, her rambling might well have been the result of the severe pain she must have been experiencing because of her stomach cancer and possibly the cancer having spread to her brain. Her misdiagnosis, subsequent mistreatment and the trauma of finding herself in a mental asylum could have only added to her misery.

Annie's case was not an isolated one. In the same year, another younger woman, 'Bridget', aged thirty-one, was admitted to the Cork Asylum because she was suicidal. Bridget had no occupation and had only been married for eleven months when her husband left her. She was described as a silent, quiet woman with a vacant look, thin and emaciated, 'tore at her dresses' and could 'become cross, abusive and depressed'. Bridget was put to work in the laundry and, since she was losing weight, was given 'two extra pints of milk'. Her bodily health must have been causing some concern as the chaplain had set aside three pounds for her burial. She was eventually transferred to hospital, where it was found that she had cancer with an enlarged gland in the right breast discharging puss. Dr Townsend refused to carry out an operation as the patient was too emaciated and the cancerous growth was too deep. By 1899 Bridget was dying. Her abdomen was dense and hard and her bowels were so obstructed that even an enema or purgatives could not relieve them. Cancer of the bowel was suspected. On the morning of 4 March 1899 Bridget died aged thirty-five. Nothing in her notes suggested that she was in any way mad.

What lay behind these admissions can only be explained by a series of errors. These cases appear to be have been misdiagnoses of physical symptoms, something that has been common for decades. In the Victorian era, hysterical girls and women were believed to present with physical symptoms which were, in fact, produced in response to an hysterical reaction to a difficult emotion. It was therefore unsurprising that when a female complained of pain or other symptoms that the doctors could not explain, they could be deemed 'hysterical' or mentally ill.

A further, more clear-cut case of 'misdiagnosis' was that of a 22-year-old labourer's daughter who was admitted to the Cork Asylum in April 1894 as suicidal. She had attempted to cut her own throat and to jump out of a window. The young woman, 'Marian', was said to have a 'morbid condition of brain' but declared physically fit although it turned out that she had not been menstruating for at least three months. Marian was pregnant, probably, according to her notes, by a farm boy she had been seeing five months previously. Her pregnancy was the obvious cause of her distress, a case of mental anguish causing physical affects which resulted in her having fits of hysteria. Having a baby out of wedlock in nineteenth-century Ireland brought disgrace on the woman and her whole family. The teaching of Catholic moral theology that sexual intercourse was for the procreation of children within the sacrament of marriage meant that a child born outside wedlock was conceived in sin. Her suicide attempts were not, in fact, a result of mental illness at all but a consequence of the shame brought on by the thought of bearing an illegitimate child. It would have been almost impossible for a Catholic unmarried mother from rural Ireland to keep her child at this time because of the amount of stigma involved and the destitution she and her baby would suffer with no help from the state. In August 1894, she gave birth to a baby boy but nothing more was written about the child. Marian was then diagnosed as suffering from a lung problem but was discharged soon after, described as 'recovered'. We can only surmise what happened to the baby and indeed Marian when she was discharged from the asylum as the Cork foundling hospital was closed in 1855 and replaced by the Union Workhouse which had opened in 1840. There were few institutions for destitute children and a pregnant girl or unmarried mother would often take her own or her baby's life because she was unable to face the shame or the poverty brought about by an illegitimate child. Employment for a single woman with a baby would have been virtually impossible, so if her family would not help her (and most parents disowned their daughter in this situation), both Marian and her baby probably ended up in the workhouse.

In his manual, *Insanity and Allied Neuroses* (1884), physician George Savage provided a chapter on the causes of insanity in which he included a few physical instigators of mental illness. Some of the reasons listed were domestic trouble, adverse circumstances, mental anxiety, overwork, religious excitement, love affairs (including seduction), fright and nervous shock. He ignored the pain caused by a corporeal illness such as cancer, as seen in the cases above, or the suffering caused both physically and mentally by a sexually transmitted disease.[14] However, he recorded, 'Exciting cases may, like predisposing ones be either psychical or physical. Mental disorder may equally be produced by a mental shock or a blow to the head.'[15] Savage admitted that the reason for mental illness might be uniform or multiform in nature, adding, 'I would say, in fact, that one cause may be predisposing and exciting,[16] or exciting alone; that there are causes which may be considered as complex or mixed, and that some causes act both physically and morally.'[17] This attitude covered multiple reasons for a person being admitted to a mental asylum and helped to demonstrate how so many women with physical ailments ended up being treated for insanity. Both medical texts and patients' records show that being female in the nineteenth century was a cause for concern in itself; their nature and their biology were perceived as leaving them far more vulnerable to psychological illness than men. It is not surprising therefore that when a woman presented with unexplained symptoms, she would often be diagnosed as hysterical or as suffering from some type of mania rather than having her physical illness be properly detected.

In October 1862, Dr John Charles Bucknill[18] wrote an article entitled *Modes of Death Prevalent among Insane*,[19] in which he called for consistency in the way causes of death were recorded in asylums. Bucknill found that the term 'exhaustion' was used vaguely in a manner that gave little clue as to the actual disease or condition that caused the patient's death. He gave the example of a male patient who, similar to Susannah Downing, had refused food because of his delusions and, like Susannah, was recorded as having died from exhaustion. Bucknill urged doctors to be more specific about what happened and he wrote: 'Let us say that the patient died of acute mania, or acute melancholia', adding, 'if we think fit, that the mode of death was anemic syncope from refusal of food'.

During the nineteenth century, certain infectious diseases were known to leave the sufferer with lasting physical disfigurement. Women were believed to be particularly affected by the facial scars of such illnesses as smallpox and scarlet fever which could change their appearance, reduce their self-esteem and lower their chances of marriage. Vaccination against smallpox was developed by Jenner in 1798, and in 1840, the Vaccination Act made it compulsory for all infants under six months to be vaccinated against smallpox; a further act in 1867 increased the age of compulsory vaccination to between six months and fourteen years. This would, eventually, lead the diminution of the disease. However, in the mid-nineteenth century there were serious outbreaks of smallpox and scarletina (scarlet fever) in London and the working-class poor were more susceptible to infection because of the close proximity of other people due to high density housing. The affect that 'pockmarks', the scarring left by smallpox, or other forms of skin disfigurement, could have on mental health did not appear to register with doctors who were mainly concerned with those who were actively suffering with infection.[20]

Despite the lack of perception by the Victorian alienists, some literary figures of the day had already made the connection between facial disfigurement and mental illness. Charles Dickens had understood the life-changing consequences that smallpox scarring had on Esther Summerson in *Bleak House* or the effects a disfiguring lip scar had on Rosa Dartle in *David Copperfield*. Similarly, in real life, Elizabeth Batte, a patient in Colney Hatch from 1854, had a physical disfigurement, possibly caused by scarlet fever, which resulted in mental disturbance and was the foundation of a wasted life. She was thirty-seven, single, literate and a housekeeper. Because she was suicidal, her condition was put down to mental anxiety and overwork. She had suffered some sort of breakdown before and had been ensconced in the Peckham asylum. In her second episode, she imagined that she had a 'snake twisted around her body' and had an 'uncontrollable desire for suicide'. She was recorded as having a chronic disease of the skin, possibly the result of scarlet fever, which, as previously mentioned, was a very common and life-threatening disease in the nineteenth century, however, Elizabeth's notes do not make it clear whether she had the fever in childhood or as an adult. One of the main symptoms of scarlet fever is a very high temperature; if she had suffered this for a lengthy period, it is possible that she might have also suffered some brain damage. Her 'disease of the skin' might also have been caused by scarlet fever as it instigated drying and peeling of the skin which could cause or exacerbate chronic skin conditions such as eczema. Her mother said that her daughter could be violent without provocation. Elizabeth was also said to be suffering from 'disappointment' which was not specified but usually referred to unrequited love. By the time Elizabeth went to Colney Hatch it would seem that she was depressed, tired and needed tranquillity. She was recorded as melancholy, peaceful and anxious to be taken care of in the asylum; her thoughts of suicide appear to have receded.

Elizabeth's notes restarted in 1862 when she would have been forty-five. From 1862 to 1864, all that was written about her was that she was 'maniacal, deluded and occasionally violent'. This picture did not fit with the description of the younger Elizabeth and by 1871 she was said to be 'excitable', a general term used by Victorian mind doctors, employed to describe various different states of mind in which the patient was not completely calm. This could have meant that her mania had become less extreme or that she was somewhat hysterical. Despite her excitability, Elizabeth was seen as a 'useful needlewoman' so it could be deduced from this observation that she was not constantly agitated but had her moments of quiet work. By 1881 a change had occurred and Elizabeth had become 'very fanciful': she refused to use any article that had been used by other patients and demanded everything 'fresh from the stores'. She lived on the 'nineteenth spur', possibly one of the female wards that jutted out from the main building, and never went 'North' of it. By the time Elizabeth reached sixty-five, she had been in the asylum for twenty-eight years and had become completely institutionalized. Although a 'cheerful old dame', she cultivated solitary habits to such a degree as to never associate with any patient in the ward. She read light literature and was said to be still in good bodily health. The only suggestion that she might still have some mental problems was found in the assertion that she would rave at times if she did not have her own way. In 1884 Elizabeth's notes reported, 'She is visited daily by the Medical Superintendent, who is her only medical advisor, custom having dictated that the assistant medical officer is not required'. She was bright and sensible in her conversation, 'altho lonely and solitary in her habits', quite a recluse living in her own room and doing her own cooking, washing and cleaning. She was on 'two chops a day with egg and two ounces of brandy'. She was said to have 'occasional flooding from the womb' and her health was slightly impaired thereby. She had continued with her needlework, making all the diapers[21] for the use of the female patients but had not been out of the ward for years. By the time Elizabeth was sixty-seven it was her physical rather than her mental health that was cause for concern. She was now visited daily by the medical superintendent rather than by the assistant medical officer. In January 1894 she had an accidental fall and fractured her seventh right rib, which heralded a decline in Elizabeth's physical health. In June she was still in bed even though the rib had mended. She only got up occasionally and complained of pain in the area of the fracture. By December that year she was recorded as 'hypocondriacal'. Suddenly it seems that Elizabeth had once more been diagnosed as having simply a mental illness because she was complaining about being in pain. In March 1895 her psychological state had once more become more important than her physical and it was noted that there was no mental improvement and her health was impaired. Two years later, aged eighty, Elizabeth died from 'exhaustion of dementia, heart disease and chronic bronchitis'. A poignant note on Elizabeth's death certificate read, 'Friend – H Bonnet, 4 Paris Gardens, Bayswater'. After forty-three years in Colney Hatch she had no family, just the mention of a friend of whom we know nothing, not even if she, or he, visited Elizabeth in the asylum. Whether this was a case of physical illness being misinterpreted as being mental is unclear, as it is complicated. What is apparent, with hindsight, was the ease with which the doctors had put Elizabeth's pain down to hypochondria and seemingly ignored the possibility that her mental distress could initially have been due to a real, physical ailment, the disfigurement of her skin.

Anorexia

Female patients who were diagnosed with religious mania frequently tried to take their own lives by refusing to eat and those who believed that they had transgressed the will of God would punish themselves so that God would forgive them; so religious mania and anorexia were closely associated. Women were often guided by auditory hallucinations to starve themselves in order to gain mercy from God not only for themselves but for all mankind. This behaviour was similar to that of the 'Holy Anorexic' described by Rudolph Bell in his book of the same name.[22]

When she was seventeen, Esther Whibley believed that she had done something to offend God, yet she was still tormented by her 'unpardonable sin' at twenty-nine, when in 1860 she was admitted to Bethlem suffering from 'religious excitement'. Esther was described as sober, having a good education and her religion as 'Independent'. She was suicidal, having tried to kill herself twice, believing that she had ruined her family by her misconduct and her soul was lost forever. Esther refused food and, according to her mother, had 'endeavoured to terminate her existence' by stuffing her handkerchief down her throat and by tightly tying her garter around her neck. She was discharged a year after her admittance to Bethlem and all that was noted was that she was 'uncured'. Whether a life-changing event was the catalyst for Esther's madness was not mentioned in her records, nor was the treatment she received. One treatment that was recommended for cases where the patient refused to eat was forced feeding. In 1868, Henry Maudsley advised this as a 'last resort' when physical health was compromised by lack of nutrition: 'Where there is a persistent refusal of food, it must never be allowed to continue so as to endanger the bodily health; and if persuasion and perseverance entirely fail, then the stomach pump must be used to administer food.'[23]

Women used religion and religious imagery when giving a reason for self-starvation, punishing themselves for their sinfulness by refusing food. Sara Ann Stoody, an unmarried dressmaker, believed that the Devil was coming to take her away. She thought that she had 'lost all her love from her heart', could not pray and did not care for her parents any more. She felt that she was being consumed in a fire, and she refused to eat so that she could die more quickly. Sara Ann's depression and her suicidal thoughts could only articulate her feelings through the medium of a biblical language and religious teaching.

Anorexia nervosa was named as a specific condition in 1873 by Dr William Withey Gull, physician to Queen Victoria, even though fasting and self-starving were hardly new phenomena.[24] It was seen as a form of female hysteria by many Victorian mad doctors and has been explained in numerous different ways since. One explanation was that anorexia reflected the nineteenth-century attitude towards the repression of women who tried to take back control by their refusal of food. However, this theory seemed to have been relevant only to middle- and upper-class girls. Women in the county asylums who rejected food did not do so as a protest against their lot nor to become the Victorian image of the pale, wasting girl languishing on the sofa in a peculiarly feminine role,[25] rather they would not eat because either they wanted to die or they believed that their food was poisoned. They wished to leave this world because it was too painful for them to go on living and this pain was a punishment from God.

It was not only Christian women who interpreted their illness through religion. The Old Testament and ideas about the God of Wrath also played an important part in the psyche of Jewish women. One case was that of Rosetta Hirshfeld, a 21-year-old Jewish woman who 'helped in a shop'. During the year prior to her illness she had been doing a great deal of heavy and laborious work, despite the fact that she was very delicate, had suffered from convulsions in her infancy and childhood, and had been diagnosed with slight lateral curvature of the spine. In May 1870, her father noticed that she had become 'very queer' in her conversation and behaviour. She said that she was an angel and that she could see the Queen asking to be admitted into heaven. At the same time, she told her father not to touch her, for if he did, he would go at once to hell. Rosetta suddenly refused to eat and at this point in her notes two pieces of information were added in an attempt to explain her condition; her brother was similarly affected, and from her childhood she had experienced difficulty in emptying her bladder. The inclusion of this information made Rosetta's condition compatible with nineteenth-century thinking on the physical and hereditary causes of mental illness. She was admitted to Bethlem and after three days was absolutely refusing to take food and was being force-fed with the stomach pump. She was said to be weak and emaciated and that her mental condition was that of acute mania. Ten days following her admittance to the asylum, Rosetta was still being fed with the stomach pump and was becoming physically weaker. After receiving treatment for just seventeen days, she died, her death not attributed to her refusal to eat but to acute mania and spinal disease. Why Rosetta starved herself to death went unexplained, but what we do know is that she chose to use religious symbolism in order to explain and control her situation and ultimately free herself from her misery.

Anorexia is usually identified as being a young woman's disorder; however, according to asylum case books, it was not only young girls who used the refusal of food as their method of committing suicide. Elizabeth Hearne, the wife of a labourer, was sixty when she was taken into Fairmile Hospital in Berkshire in 1872, suffering from melancholia and religious delusions. She believed that she held conversations with the Devil and that he had taken her soul. Because she felt that there was no hope for her, Elizabeth tried to drown herself in the bath but failed. In her notes it said that she eventually died in 1873 as a result of exhaustion from melancholia and refusal of food. Suicidal tendencies and actual attempts as the result of a belief that they were lost to God were common amongst women. When the urge to kill themselves became overpowering, they believed that they were in the power of the Devil who was urging them to do themselves harm.

Female sexuality

Overt, or what was perceived as depraved, sexuality in women was seen as a symptom of many categories of female insanity. Its manifestation at any stage of the female life cycle could lead to incarceration, even when no other symptoms were present. It is because of this that we can find asylum inmates such as Priscilla Hennessy, the twenty-year-old single daughter of an upholsterer who, in 1860, was put into Bethlem because she was found to be masturbating.

Although nineteenth-century doctors did not always agree over the aetiology of nervous diseases, they often treated the symptoms with their particular medical model whilst attributing the women's suffering to internal biological factors associated with the womb. Some of these 'treatments' could be extremely violent. Dr W. Tyler Smith, one of the founders of the Obstetrical Society in 1859, wrote about treatments suggested for the erotic and nervous symptoms of the menopause. He recommended a course of injections of ice water into the rectum, the introduction of ice into the vagina and leeching of the labia and the cervix. He wrote, with what seems to be a sense of admiration for the leeches, 'The suddenness with which the leeches applied to this part fill themselves considerably increases the good effects of their application and for some hours after their removal there is an oozing of blood from their leech bites.'[26] According to Smith, 'The death of the reproductive faculty (during the menopause) is accompanied ... by struggles which implicate every organ and every function of the body.'[27]

One of Smith's contemporaries who wrote about the causes of insanity was Sir Alexander Morison (1779–1866), who was consultant physician at Bethlem Hospital. He too had specific ideas about women who were experiencing the menopause and said that the change of life frequently led to periods of insanity.[28] Robert Brudnell Carter believed that the suppression of emotion, particularly sexual passion, was observed more frequently in women than in men. This was because he believed that women had to discipline their feelings more, 'That these derangements are much more common in the female than in the male, women not only being more prone to emotions, but also more frequently under the necessity of endeavouring to conceal them.'[29] He noted:

If relative power of emotion against the sexes be compared in the present day, even without including the erotic passion, it is seen to be considerably greater in the woman than in the man, partly from natural conformation which causes the former to feel, under circumstances where the latter thinks; and partly because the woman is more under the necessity of endeavouring to conceal her feelings. But when sexual desire is taken into account, it will add immensely to the forces bearing upon the female, who is often much under its dominion and who if unmarried and chaste is compelled to restrain every manifestation of its sway.[30]

Carter's theory that admitted that women had sexual desires and feelings differed from many other Victorian doctors who believed that these physical needs were the prerogative of men only. William Acton (1813–1875), doctor, gynaecologist and writer who was well known for his views on masturbation, wrote in his book on the functions and disorders of the reproductive system:

I should say that the majority of women (happily for them) are not very much troubled with sexual feeling of any kind. What men are habitually, women are only exceptionally. It is too true, I admit, as the divorce courts show, that there are some few women who have sexual desires so strong that they surpass those of men. … I admit, of course the existence of sexual excitement terminating even in nymphomania, a form of insanity, which those accustomed to visit lunatic asylums, must be fully conversant with.[31]

Sexual passion could sometimes be found in the 'fallen woman' whose desires had been aroused by experiencing intercourse, but, according to Acton, the best mothers and managers of households only felt passion for their children, their home and their domestic duties. A modest woman should submit to her husband to gratify his sexual desires, not hers. It should be the wish to have children that really made a married woman have sex with her husband; otherwise she would have rather been relieved from his attentions. Mistresses and prostitutes were considered to be the class of women who actually enjoyed sexual intercourse. When it was found to be the case that sexual feelings were present in a woman, she could be made subject to horrendous physical abuse in the name of psychiatric intervention.

Isaac Baker Brown (1811–1873), published a work, *On the Curability of Certain Forms of Insanity, Epilepsy, Catalepsy, and Hysteria in Females* (1866). He was a prominent gynaecologist and obstetrical surgeon, was one of the founders of St. Mary's Hospital in London and was to become the president of the Medical Society of London in 1865. He would later have his work discredited and be expelled from the Obstetrical Society of London in 1867 for carrying out operations on patients who did not or could not give their consent. In setting out his theory for the onset of insanity in many females, masturbation, along with its cure, clitoridectomy, Brown listed sixteen 'gentlemen' who, amongst very many others, had been led to adopt his views.[32] He believed:

> Every medical practitioner must have met with a certain class of cases which has set at defiance every effort at diagnosis, baffled every treatment, and belied every prognosis. ... The patient becomes restless and excited, or melancholy and retiring; listless and indifferent to the social influences of domestic life. She will be fanciful in her food, sometimes express even a distaste for it, and apparently (as her friends will say) live upon nothing. She will always be ailing, and complaining of different affections. At first, perhaps, dyspepsia and sickness will be observed; then pain in the head and down the spine; pain more or less constant, in the lower part of the back, or on either side in the lumbar region. There will be wasting of the face and muscles generally; the skin sometimes becomes dry and harsh, at other times cold and clammy.[33]

To these so-called 'physical evidences of derangement', Brown added several gynaecological problems in the cases of single females along with a distaste for marital intercourse in married women. He wrote that if these symptoms were left unchecked then they could lead to more serious consequences, 'The patient either becomes a confirmed invalid, always ailing, and confined to bed or sofa, or, on the other hand, will become subject to catalepsy, epilepsy, idiocy, or insanity.'[34] These physical symptoms could have easily been the indicators of bodily illness; even life-threatening conditions, as was observed in the case of Sarah Rebecca Thorley whose consumption was seemingly misdiagnosed as hysteria, were brought on by masturbation. Sarah was admitted to Colney Hatch Asylum in November 1859 and she remained a patient there until her death in 1865. She was diagnosed as suffering from dementia, a strange judgement as she was only twenty-eight, but at this time dementia was used to describe many different conditions that included some form of intellectual deficit. The term was applied to psychotic illnesses which were thought to have a dementing process and had behavioural connotations. Henry Monro (1817–1891), the noted mad doctor, said in 1856 that dementia should always be applied to a passive rather than an active state.[35]

Before her admission to the asylum, Sarah worked as a governess which implied that she had a reasonable level of education. She was described as being 'violent, hysterical, pale and suffering from memory lapses', as well as, 'demented, idle, slovenly' but in fair bodily health. She could not even remember the death of her own mother. She occasionally played on the piano but wandered from one time to another distractedly. Sarah was reportedly 'of dirty habits' and would not wear any night dress but lay between the sheets in a 'state of nudity'. Her 'dirty habits' was a reference to masturbation as it was recorded that Sarah habitually stimulated her sexual organs. In the nineteenth century, masturbation was regarded as an immoral practice, often referred to as 'dirty habits' in asylum medical notes. It was reported to have caused all sorts of mental and physical disabilities, including epilepsy, consumption, infertility, hysteria and fits.[36] It was seen as being morally reprehensible and physically debilitating causing ailments such as memory loss, paralysis and imbecility. The acknowledgement that women and girls could indulge themselves in this way was a rejection of the Victorian ideals of female modesty and purity. Following a gap of six years in Sarah's notes, it was documented that she had died on the morning of Sunday 12 March 1865 from gradual exhaustion caused by pulmonary consumption yet Sarah had been suffering from illness for several years. By the time she died, she was far from being in 'fair bodily health' as noted on her admittance; in fact she was recorded as being emaciated. In what seemed to be some sort of attempt to mitigate the seriousness of the situation, she was said to have refused all medication or to wear flannel or warm dress but liked to read books of a religious tendency.

One interesting comment about Sarah Thorley was that she did not show much affection for her sisters and preferred the company of her fellow patients to that of the nurses or other sane persons.

A letter, found tucked into the casebook with Sarah's notes, made chilling reading and could account for this pitiable young woman's so-called dementia and lack of regard for her family. It was written by Dr D Fraser Marshall Sgn. From 15 Harrington Square, London N.W. on 5 November 1859, when Sarah was sent to Colney Hatch Asylum[37]:

Dear Sir,

Yesterday I signed a certificate of insanity in the case of Miss S.R. Thorley, previous to her removal to Colney Hatch – there is one circumstance connected with her condition, which you ought to know, as it will guide you in adopting the treatments most likely to be beneficial – the fact was related to me by Mr. Healy, in consequence of which I questioned Miss Thorley's sister, and learnt from her that at an early age (9 or 10 years) the patient, being under the evil influence of a worthless maidservant, contracted the vicious habits of self indulgence which have increased with her years; an operation, the excision of part of the clitoris, was performed, but without any apparent benefit.

Faithfully yours,

D Fraser Marshall sgn.

It was common for the children of the Victorian middle classes to be cared for by servants who were from a completely different order from their charges and were therefore deemed to have looser sexual morals. Many of these servants were single, young women who frequently cared for the young children in the household where they were employed and usually spent a lot of time with them. Upper- and middle-class ladies with infants or toddlers would not care for the physical needs of their children but would delegate these tasks to a maid or a nurse. It therefore fell to a servant of inferior class to feed, change, pot, discipline and put to bed small children. Because of their close, physical proximity to their little charges, these servant girls and women were often the ones who first awakened sexual feelings in the child.[38]

In her observations on class and gender in Victorian England, Leonora Davidoff was principally talking about the relationship between nursemaids and their male charges, but it must have been easy to lay the blame on a 'worthless maidservant' when a little girl, the daughter of middle-class parents, was found to be masturbating. Female masturbation was an unmentionable subject in the nineteenth century although male masturbation was frequently written about and was believed by some doctors to lead to madness. In 1861, John Millar, writing on the dangers of masturbation said of girls, 'Though nymphomanic symptoms are constantly present when young females are insane, I have met with only one instance in which I could say that the mental disturbance was due to this vice; and this patient continues in a hopeless state of dementia.'[39] At this time, nymphomania was believed to be a specific organic disease, classifiable, with an assumed set of symptoms, causes and treatments. It was sometimes described as too much sexual desire and too much masturbation.

The idea of a young girl undergoing a clitoridectomy in Victorian times was not unusual. Surgeon Fraser Marshall described his procedure as 'the excision of part of the clitoris'; Dr Isaac Baker Brown recommended its complete removal to prevent masturbation. However, historians such as Lesley Hall believe that there is little evidence that this procedure was ever a routine prescription for Victorian medical men.[40] It had gained temporary notoriety through the activities of Baker Brown, who was an advocate and practitioner of it in the 1860s. This may have been the case, yet the discovery of Dr Marshall's letter concerning Sarah Thorley could signify that this was a more common procedure than previously presumed by historians. Indeed, one of the Scottish lunatic asylums had recorded occasional instances of the procedure to curb habitual masturbation.[41]

Whatever had happened to Sarah Thorley when she was a young girl, by the age of twenty-eight she was in an asylum having been certified as mad when she was suffering from pulmonary consumption. The symptoms of her perceived madness were, however, also symptoms of tuberculosis: night sweats (she refused to wear a nightdress), fatigue (she was idle and slovenly) and confusion (she was distracted and forgetful). It was hardly surprising that Sarah was not affectionate towards her sisters as she probably rejected her family together with all medical staff following her treatment. Perhaps Sarah read religious books in an attempt to discover some meaning for her present life or hope for peace in a future one.

It was not extraordinary to discover that women with grave physical illnesses could be viewed as suffering from mental ill health and treated accordingly. In some cases, this meant that they followed a regime of rest, nourishment and mild occupation that would not have cured their illness but would not have exacerbated it either. For those unfortunate women, like Rebecca Thorley, who found themselves in the hands of Isaac Baker Brown or one of his fellow practitioners, there could have been a much more painful and damaging outcome. This was further demonstrated in Baker Brown relating the treatment of some of his hysteria cases.

Case 1, 1859: Brown said that the patient, referred to as D.E., had been ill for five years and was cured, by his intervention, in two months. She was a single, 26-year-old dressmaker from Yorkshire who had been unable to work for five years and was being supported by her former customers. D.E. was very thin and weak, was always sick after meals, was in great pain and suffered from chronic acidity. She had constant burning, aching pain in her lower back. Her periods were irregular; she had heavy vaginal discharge and was constipated. D.E. was melancholy and wanted to be cured. Brown's reaction to this patient was that: 'Her physiognomy at once told me the nature of the case.' He advised her admittance to hospital where he carried out his first operation where he 'divided the clitoris subcutaneously'. Baker Brown believed that the 'unnatural irritation' of the clitoris caused epilepsy, hysteria and mania, so he advocated removing or partially removing it in patients whom he suspected of masturbating. Case 1 was Brown's first attempt in proving his theory; however, clitoridectomy as a method of depriving a female of sexual pleasure was not a new idea. It is not known exactly when the practice started although some historians believe that it has been traced back to ancient Egypt.

Baker Brown's operations for hysteria were carried out in the following manner on females over ten years old. The patient was given a warm bath and a clearance of the portal circulation. She was then put completely under the influence of chloroform and her clitoris was excised by scissors or a knife; Brown favoured the use of scissors. When this had been completed, the wound was plugged with graduated compresses of lint and a pad, well secured by T bandages. A grain of opium was introduced per rectum. The patient was then placed in bed and carefully watched by a nurse to prevent haemorrhage by any disturbance of the dressing. The patient had a prescribed diet that must be unstimulating. It consisted of milk, farinaceous food, fish and occasionally chicken; all alcoholic or fermented liquors were strictly forbidden. D.E. was unfortunate because her operation was followed by profuse haemorrhaging and opiates had to be used to help her to sleep. She had olive oil rubbed into her chest and she followed the recommended diet which was free from any stimulants. According to Brown, D.E. was better within two months of the operation and was able to return to her occupation. We only have his word for this, along with the assertion that she remained well for six years.

Isaac Baker Brown claimed many such cures following his 'usual operation' and he listed the cases in his work on the curability of certain forms of insanity. When Emma K., a single, 22-year-old woman was admitted to the London Surgical Home in 1863, she had been ill for many years. At sixteen she suffered from piles, which 'occasioned very much irritation and pain after each evacuation, aggravated by constipation and walking'. She had heavy periods which lasted for eight days and had been under long and varied medical treatment, without benefit. On examination, Brown found evidence of masturbation, although he does not say what evidence this was. Often an enlarged clitoris was thought to be a sure sign of masturbation. He therefore performed his operation which he recorded, yet again, as successful. The proof was seen in the fact that three years later, Emma married and gave birth to a living child; her 'cure' was attributed to marriage and progeny, the allotted purpose in life for a Victorian woman.

It would seem that Brown used his operations to ideological ends as well as in the hope that he was alleviating the symptoms of hysteria. When he saw Mrs O, he reported that since her marriage five years previously, she had been ill, having distaste for the society of her husband. She always lay upon the sofa and was under medical treatment. Brown found 'evidence of peripheral excitement'[42] and operated on her. She rapidly lost all her hysterical symptoms and, a year later, 'came up to town to consult me concerning a tumour, which greatly frightened her, as she feared it was ovarian'. There was no tumour; the 'lady' was six months pregnant and two years later she had her second child. Mrs O had been diagnosed as ill and sterile. Following her operation her cure was complete with the added benefit of pregnancy and two children. Brown had, according to his case studies, restored Mrs O to robust health and the acceptable state of motherhood.

One of Baker Brown's most disturbing cases concerned a twenty-year-old woman who had been confined to a spinal couch since she was fourteen because she indulged in masturbation that allegedly left her debilitated. She was made to wear 'a spinal apparatus, attached to which was a steel spring pressing on sacrum and pubis, and intended to support the perinaeum and keep the uterus in position'. Brown made his usual diagnosis, 'The cause of spinal irritation, or paresis, may be defined in one word – "debility"; this debility always, or almost always, being due to inhibitory irritation'. 'The state of things may give rise to wide and varied disorders, all the symptoms of which are asthenic in their character and all of which are marked by extreme nervous prostration.'

'Without doubt, – for all authors agree on this point, one of the most prominent causes is peripheral irritation of the pubic nerve, producing undue exhaustion.'[43] However, his methods were strongly contested as the young woman was very religious. It was also thought that his operation might interfere with her eventual marital happiness and even prevent procreation. To Brown, these objections were untenable, even though he admitted that he could not cite actual cases to contradict the fears expressed. He was finally permitted to perform his operation and although there were some setbacks he said that after a month, 'This lady was able to walk three miles.'

Elaine Showalter wrote: 'The rise of the Victorian madwoman was one of history's self-fulfilling prophecies.'[44] To be a female was to be childlike, irrational and sexually unstable with a nervous and reproductive system that made her particularly vulnerable to mental instability. Coupled with the fact that women were also legally powerless, such attitudes could and did lead male doctors to some unreasonable diagnoses and horrific 'cures'. The nineteenth century was associated with the more humane treatment of the insane as the idea of moral management offered the promise of cure through kindness and persuasion. This may have been beneficial to some women who were incarcerated in asylums due to their being physically ill, as they would have, at least, received rest and nourishment. However, as we have observed, this was not always the case and many women suffered and died in terrible, unrecognized pain[45] or were left to the mercy of doctors who used sexual mutilation to control, what they believed to be, the cause of women's hysteria.

Asylums and Madness Mirrored in Nineteenth-Century Literature

I really believe my nerves are getting over-stretched: my mind has suffered
somewhat too much; a malady is growing upon it – what shall I do? How
shall I keep well?

Lucy Snowe in *Villette* chapter 15.

The contemporary understanding of madness and the workings of asylums, by both doctors and society in general, were reflected in nineteenth-century literature. Portrayals of madwomen frequently saw them as unfeminine, wild and murderous and contrary to the Victorian ideal of femininity. Lunacy was often revealed as an inherited condition usually passed from mother to daughter. Female novelists and poets were more understanding of the reasons behind perceived mental illness, especially those who had felt the deprivations, constrictions and loneliness experienced by many nineteenth-century women.

Imaginative literary texts articulated the inner turmoil experienced by many Victorian women, allowing female novelists to express a certain freedom in fiction. In doing so, they avoided the danger of personal exposure of their own thoughts and feelings on the subject. Charlotte Brontë's *Villette* (1853), for example, presented the disturbances of the young female mind in its social context. Its heroine, Lucy Snowe, suffers from extreme loneliness and depression; without close friends or family, she has to find her way through a world that was unsympathetic to the single, penniless woman. Her isolation, lack of true love or friendship and hard work caused her to suffer from nervous exhaustion and psychological trauma, even though doctors at this time were inclined to blame menstrual disorders or sexual abnormality as the main cause for women's mental breakdowns.

Portrayals of women's madness in Victorian literature will be explored in this chapter to illustrate how they reflected contemporary fear and understanding of insanity. The principal works chosen are: Mrs Gaskell's *Ruth* (1853), *The Poor Clare* (1856) and *Cousin Phillis* (1864); Charles Dickens's *Great Expectations* (1861); Rosina Bulwer Lytton's *A Blighted Life* (1880); Charlotte Brontë's *Jane Eyre* (1847) and *Villette* (1853); Mary Elizabeth Braddon's *Lady Audley's Secret* (1861–1862); Mrs Henry Wood's *St. Martin's Eve* (1885); Gustave Flaubert's *Madame Bovary* (1856); and Wilkie Collins's *The Woman in White* (1860). Authors often had personal experience of mental ill health through their own experience or that of friends and family. Charles Dickens was interested in psychology and the treatment of the insane. Amongst his close acquaintants in the early 1850s was the psychiatrist John Connolly and this friendship, no doubt, gave him insight into an insider's opinion on female madness, influencing his fiction. In *Great Expectations*, Miss Havisham displays realistic and precise symptoms of hysterical insanity as classified by Conolly.[1] In *Little Dorrit* (1855–1857), Maggy, the mentally retarded young woman and Miss Wade, who was consumed with anger and jealousy due to her lowly position as a governess, are well drawn and Mrs Jellaby in *Bleak House* (1852–1853) shows symptoms of monomania as she is fixated on good causes, to the detriment of her family. Her husband is driven to thoughts of suicide.

Literature written around the same period by different authors provided relevant vision into ideas of female madness. Emily Dickinson (1830–1886) dramatized interior schisms suffered by women in her poem, 'One Need Not Be a Chamber to Be Haunted'. Her work shows the complicated psychological state in which many women found themselves:

> One need not be a chamber to be haunted,
> One need not be a house;
> The brain has corridors surpassing
> Material place.

> Far safer, of a midnight meeting
> External ghost,
> Than an interior confronting
> That whiter host ....

Dickinson expresses the idea of the buried self in a frightening and haunting way:

> Ourself, behind ourself, concealed,
> Should startle most;
> Assassin, hid in our apartment,
> Be horror's least.

The last stanza in the poem echoes the subject of a short story written by Mrs Gaskell called *The Poor Clare*. In *The Poor Clare*, Lucy has been placed under a curse so that she is outwardly gentle, feminine and kind whilst within she is 'a horror', a devil. Lucy, and at times those around her, can physically perceive this inner, buried self: 'In the great mirror opposite I saw myself, and right behind another wicked, fearful self, so like me that my soul seemed to quiver within me, as though not knowing to which similitude of body it belonged.' At this vision Lucy swooned and whilst in bed, her double was seen by all, 'flitting about the house and gardens about some mischievous or detestable work'. Mrs Gaskell, posing the question, 'Yet this sounded like the tale of one bewitched; or was it merely the effect of extreme seclusion telling on the nerves of a sensitive girl?'[2] shows her insight into the workings of the mind.

Stories of Victorian, working-class girls falling prey to men of a higher social status than them were well documented by historians and writers of literary fiction. This genre of nineteenth-century literature was, to a large extent, reflected in the treatment of women who were rejected in love. Their lack of power and status accounted for their seduction and abandonment. In *Ruth* (1853), Ruth, an innocent, naïve, young orphan girl is seduced by an aristocratic man and becomes pregnant. When she is abandoned by her lover, she attempts suicide. She reaches the depths of despair because she has lost the man who she believed to be in love with her and she is ostracized for being a fallen woman. In *Cousin Phillis* (1864), Gaskell tells the story of Phillis, a country girl innocent of the ways of the world, who falls in love with her cousin's boss, Mr Holdsworth, a well-travelled, urbane dandy. When Holdsworth stays with Phillis and her parents on their farm whilst he is recuperating from an illness, he falls for Phillis but does not tell her so. When he is sent to Canada to set up a railway line, he reveals his feelings to Phillis' cousin, Paul Manning, and tells him that he intends to return when he has made some money and a name for himself, and ask Phillis to marry him. Paul sees that his cousin is making herself ill with love for Holdsworth and decides to tell her of his proposed plans, making Phillis very happy. However, once in Canada, Holdsworth finds a new love, marries her and sends wedding cards back to his friends in England. Phillis is shattered and goes into a decline; she becomes more and more ill and behaves very strangely:

> Her hands were concealed under the table and I could see the passionate, convulsive manner in which she laced and interlaced her fingers perpetually, wringing them together from time to time, wringing till the compressed flesh became perfectly white. … her grey eyes had dark circles round them and a strange kind of dark light; her cheeks were flushed, but her lips were white and wan.[3]

This image painted by Gaskell of a young girl in the throes of extreme mental anguish mirrors the physical descriptions often found in the asylum casebooks, particularly the agitated wringing of her hands. As the passage suggests, there is worse to come when Phillis overhears her father, who sees her as a pure child and not the young woman she has become, berating cousin Paul for putting ideas into her head. Gaskell says that he did not see Phillis standing in the room until he turned his head round; then he stood still:

> She must have been half undressed; but she had covered herself with a dark winter cloak, that fell in long folds to her white, naked, noiseless feet. Her face was strangely pale: her eyes heavy in the black circles round them. She came up to the table very slowly, and leant her hand upon it, saying mournfully,
>   'Father, you must not blame Paul … I loved him father.'[4]

Her father asks her if she were not happy or loved enough at home and cannot believe that she would have left her family and gone wandering over the world with a stranger. Suddenly a shadow came over Phillis's face, and she tottered towards her father and fell down at his knees moaning: 'Father, my head! My head!' and then she slipped through his quick enfolding arms, and lay on the ground at his feet.[5] Phillis's father fears she is dead, but she is not and when the doctor arrived he diagnoses brain fever. Her hair is cut off and she has her head swathed in wet cloths and ice. Eventually she comes round but is in a deep depression. Betty, the old retainer, tells Phillis that the doctors have done all they can and now she has to fight her way back to cheerfulness or she will break her parent's hearts. In other words, she needs to pull herself together.

As Mrs Gaskell's story is fiction, Phillis follows Betty's advice and her recovery commences. She does not have to be put in an asylum. Unfortunately, stories and novels did not reflect reality to the extent that it always mirrored real life; those who were committed frequently failed to get better, as seen in the case of Sara Mumford, a 25-year-old single nurse of good education, who was admitted to Bethlem in 1855. The reason for her insanity was put down to 'disappointment in marriage'. Her notes said that she was an interesting looking girl whose mind was disordered two months before her admission due to 'disappointment in love'. She could not settle and 'walked around continuously as if looking for something'. She was discharged after three months, 'uncured'. Like Cousin Phillis, Sara was 'interesting looking', agitated and restless, but unlike her literary counterpart, she could not be restored to health.

Tess, in *Tess of the D'Urbervilles* (1891), was mentally disturbed when her son, conceived during her seduction by the wealthy, dissolute Alec, was refused Christian baptism. Thomas Hardy described Tess Durbeyfield as being 'well-grounded in the Holy Scriptures', like all village girls, and because of this 'grounding' Tess understands only too well the fate of her illegitimate child, Sorrow:

> She thought of the child consigned to the nethermost corner of hell, as its double doom for lack of baptism and lack of legitimacy; saw the arch fiend tossing it with his three pronged fork, like the one they used for heating the oven on baking days; to which picture she added many other quaint and curious details of torment sometimes taught the young in this Christian country.[6]

Tess presumably believes herself to be 'lost' as well as her son. This is made evident when, in an earlier scene, she took to heart the biblical text she witnessed being painted by a religious man whom she had stopped to talk to on her way home from Alec and the D'Urberville mansion. This particular passage read: 'Thy, Damnation, Slumbereth Not'[7] and although Tess knows she has been sinned against and tries to convince herself that God would not say such things, she nevertheless embraces the Victorian way of thinking and sees herself as lost to God:

The words entered Tess with accusatory horror. It was as if this man had known her recent history; yet he was a total stranger. ...
'Do you believe what you paint?' she asked in low tones.
'Believe that text? Do I believe in my own existence!'
'But,' she said tremulously, 'suppose your sin was not of your own seeking?'
He shook his head.
'I cannot split hairs on that burning query,' he said I have walked hundreds of miles this past summer, painting these texts on every wall, gate, and stile in the length and breadth of this district. I leave their application to the hearts of people who read 'em.'[8]

The religious man tells Tess that his texts are supposed to frighten their readers, as Tess puts it, to be 'crushing and killing'. He finds a piece of blank wall and decides to paint one that 'will be good for dangerous young females like yourself to heed'.[9] Tess turns briefly to read the first part of the inscription: 'Thou shalt not commit –' which makes her flush.

Tess was not mad in the manner depicted by most Victorian novels, but she was fearful of the loss of her soul and took the biblical texts as being directed against herself. Incisive understanding of what, in many cases, lay behind the mental health problems of numerous nineteenth-century women was only one interpretation of madness presented by Victorian writers.

'True' stories

Other novelists would concentrate on a more sensational aspect of insanity and its representation of women. Popular fiction, stimulated by outrages and the stories of real cases, drew from the world around. It derived its inspiration from newspapers, scandals, gossip and general perceptions of lunatics and madhouses. 'True' stories of people being imprisoned in mental asylums against their will were fairly common during the nineteenth century and fed the public's fear of the madhouse. Sometimes women were said to be banished to a convent asylum in Belgium or France as in the case of Lady Audley in Mary Braddon's novel of the same name. Elaine Showalter wrote: 'To find the female perspective on insanity, we must turn to Victorian women's diaries and novels.'[10] She makes the point that literature deals exclusively with the experience of middle-class and aristocratic women, yet the journals of Florence Nightingale, the psychological fiction of Charlotte Brontë and even the more sensational novels of Mary E Braddon or Wilkie Collins offer a more realistic reading of female madness than those presented by Victorian psychiatric medicine.

One exciting story that was circulating during the mid-1850s was the supposed kidnap and imprisonment of Lady Rosina Bulwer Lytton. Edward Bulwer Lytton, the well-known writer and politician, was known to be vindictive and cruel to his wife after they had split up, provoking her to write novels and letters satirizing his behaviour and further numerous letters blackening his name. In 1858, when she publicly stormed a nomination meeting on the hustings at his parliamentary constituency, denouncing her husband in front of everyone, he felt that his political career was in jeopardy and had her taken to an asylum. During this period when the scandal of Sir Edward Bulwer Lytton and his wife was appearing in the press, Wilkie Collins was writing his sensational novel, *The Woman in White*, and it was rumoured that took much of his plot from their story.

Rosina Bulwer Lytton chronicled the events surrounding her incarceration and her subsequent release a few weeks later, in a book titled *A Blighted life*. In the 'Background Story to Lady Lytton's Entrapment into an Asylum', the reader is informed that Lady Lytton and her companion Mrs Clarke made a visit to Mr Hale Thompson's House in Clarges Street London on Tuesday 21 June 1858 in order to receive an answer to the proposals she had made to her husband. It all went terribly wrong for her when she returned to the house later that day, realized that she was not going to get an answer and decided to leave the house with her friends Miss Ryves and Mrs Clarke:

> On reaching the hall we found it literally filled with two mad doctors, that fellow Hill,[11] of Inverness Lodge Brentford, his assistant, the impudent snub-nosed man who had stared so when I got out of the brougham, two women keepers, one a great thing of six feet high, the other a moderate-sized and nice looking woman, and a very idiotic-looking footman of Thompson's, with his back against the hall door to bar egress. Seeing this blockade, I exclaimed, "What a set of blackguards!" to which Mr. Hill, wagging his head, replied, "I beg you will speak like a lady, Lady Lytton."
> "I am treated so like one that I certainly ought," I answered.[12]

Following the flight of her friend Miss Ryves, and after the confrontation with her husband, who was skulking in the dining room, Lady Lytton concludes, 'nothing shall get me out of this'. As she sits in Thompson's hall the front door is opened and two policemen are brought in: 'At which, I rose to my feet and said, "Don't presume to touch me! I'll go with these vile men, but the very stones of London will rise up against them and their infamous employer".'[13] Lady Lytton is put into Hill's carriage with Hill himself, two keepers and Mrs Clarke whilst the snub-nosed assistant rode on the box. She was taken to what she refers to as Hill's 'stronghold', his private lunatic asylum, 'Inverness Lodge' in Brentford.

The journalist John Mitford, previously mentioned in Chapter 2, asserted that some women had been placed in private asylums by their husbands or other relatives in order to hide them away. Often these women were perfectly rational and sane. Mrs Scarrion had been a parlour boarder in Whitmore House Asylum for some years; this meant that she was a privileged patient whose family paid extra for her to have her own private sitting room. She was a respectable lady, accomplished, sensible and modest. Mitford claimed that her husband had confined her only because he wanted to get rid of her and that she was reconciled to her situation and looked forward to the grave as the only prospect of future happiness. Several other ladies fared worse than Mrs Scarrion because while 'in possession of reason' they were locked up with maniacs of the worst description. He said that they were shut out from all hope and unnoticed and unknown were 'bending broken hearted over an early tomb'. However, in stressing the danger these unfortunate women faced, Mitford proved himself a man of his time, espousing that the true value of a woman could only be assessed by her sexual purity and her relationship to her closest male relative:

It is not an uncommon case for female patients, married and unmarried to become pregnant by the infernal ruffians, masters and keepers, who have the care of them against whose designs and feeble barriers of separation and female keepers afford no protection. What, on recovery, must be the mental torture of a virtuous woman, the victim of these monsters, at such a retrospect? The pen drops from my hand when I think of the maddening sensation of her father – her husband.[14]

The irony that a woman's father or husband should be singled out for pity should she be assaulted when it was predominantly the male family members, father, brother, husband or even son who were responsible for the incarceration of their female relatives in mental asylums appears to have escaped him.

One case that mirrored Victorian authors' concern with false incarceration in a mental asylum was that of Caroline Brent, the 28-year-old wife of a costermonger who appeared to have been unfaithful to her husband and therefore worthy of punishment. Caroline was admitted to the Colney Hatch Asylum on 21 October 1853 said to be suffering from mania. She could read and write, was not epileptic nor was she deemed dangerous to herself or others. She had never been in an asylum before, and by the time she entered Colney Hatch she was recorded as having been insane for six weeks. According to her case notes, Caroline was deluded, she thought that she could annihilate people with her thoughts and she was subject to maniacal excitement and depression. This would seem to be a typical diagnosis and good reason for having Caroline treated in an asylum, but the letter from her husband, which was attached to her case notes, told a very different story:

> My False Hearted wife,
> I received your letter and I beg you will not mock me with "dear husband" any more. – I have had an interview with James Clark, the man you cry so much about, he has given me back some of the presents you gave him. I have also got the ring you had made for him with your hair worked in it, likewise a lock of his hair that is in your box and more things too much to name.
> I am now a miserable man for life. Were [*sic*] is a man's happiness but in his wife and home? And that you have destroyed for ever and this is what you call a little nonsense – how many men has committed suicide though [*sic*] such nonsense – I call it very series very series. [*sic*]
> So no more your much grieved and hurted husband – you proved vain hearted woman to deny your faithful husband for the sake of getting another man.

After spending just under a year in the asylum, Caroline was discharged, relieved, on 24 September 1854. Whether she was really mentally ill or considered morally insane by her husband was unknown and there are no notes to record what treatment she received.

Heredity and madness in the Victorian novel

One of the most well-known madwomen in nineteenth-century literature is Bertha Mason in *Jane Eyre*. In her depiction of this character, Charlotte Brontë employed the codified language of contemporary psychiatric discourse, in particular the way in which diagnoses were arrived at. After his aborted attempt to enter into a bigamous marriage with Jane Eyre, Rochester endeavours to justify his actions to her by explaining the background to his first marriage with Bertha Mason, his mad wife he kept prisoner in the attic of Thornfield Hall. He says that when he had left college, his father sent him out to Jamaica to: 'Espouse a bride already courted for me'.[15] He was dazzled by Bertha's beauty and married too hastily: 'A marriage was achieved almost before I knew where I was.'[16] Rochester refers to himself as a 'mole-eyed blockhead' because he had not bothered to understand his wife's true nature nor her psychological inheritance. He tells Jane:

> My bride's mother I had never seen: I understood she was dead. The honey-moon over, I learned my mistake: she was only mad; and shut up in a lunatic asylum. There was a younger brother, too; a complete dumb idiot. The elder one, whom you have seen … will probably be in the same state one day.[17]

(Rochester is referring to Richard Mason, Bertha's brother. Jane had already noted that although charming and handsome, Mason had vacant eyes and a weak face.)

When a patient was admitted into a Victorian asylum, certain observations were made, any family history of insanity being of particular importance. In his book, *The Borderlands of Insanity* (1875), Andrew Wynter noted:

> It is agreed by all alienist physicians, that girls are far more likely to inherit insanity from their mothers than from the other parent, and that the same rule obtains as regards sons. The tendency of the mother to transmit her mental disease is, however, in all cases stronger than the father's. … If the daughter of an insane mother very much resembles her in feature and in temperament, the chances are that she is more likely to inherit the disease than other daughters who are not so like. … We often see children partaking of the father's features and of the mother's temperament. In such cases the child would possibly inherit the mother's insane temperament, transmuted

into some disorder of the nervous system, such as hysteria, epilepsy, or neuralgia; for nothing is more common than to find mere nervous disorders changed, by transmission from parent to child, into mental disorders, and vice versa.[18]

Nineteenth-century mad doctors grouped hysteria, epilepsy and neuralgia together as genetically transmitted mental illnesses. The supposed likelihood that a child, especially a girl, would inherit her mother's madness was fatalistic and often used as an excuse for explaining away the real reasons for a patient's mental health problems when no other diagnosis was available. In the same way, inherited madness was used in literature to explain disturbing behaviour and to exonerate the callous attitude of characters like Mr Rochester who chose to incarcerate his wife under the care of a drunken servant.

In the case of Lady Audley in *Lady Audley's Secret*, the theory of inherited madness helped the reader understand how such a beautiful and feminine young woman could become a murderess. When Lady Audley confesses to her husband, Sir Michael, that she has killed George Talboys, her first husband, she says that she is a madwoman: 'I killed him because I AM MAD! Because my intellect is a little way upon the wrong side of the narrow boundary line between sanity and insanity.'[19] She needs to tell Sir Michael the story of her life in order for him to understand who she really is. When she was a child she would ask where her mother was as she only had a dim recollection of her. She was told that her mother was 'away' but where was a secret. She was placed in the care of a disagreeable woman whilst her father was away at sea. It was then that she learnt what it was to be poor. Eventually, in a fit of passion, Lucy Audley's foster mother revealed the truth, that her mother was in a madhouse forty miles away. Lucy immediately began to worry about her possible mental inheritance:

> I brooded horribly upon the thought of my mother's madness. It haunted me day and night. I was always picturing to myself this madwoman pacing up and down in some prison cell, in a hideous garment that bound her tortured limbs.[20]

When Lucy eventually manages to talk to her father about her mother, she discovers that he loved his wife very much and had he been able to afford to leave the navy he would have, 'willingly sacrificed his life to her, and constituted himself her guardian, had he not been compelled to earn the daily bread of the madwoman and her child by the exercise of his profession'.[21] From her father, Lucy learnt another lesson in poverty, that her mother, instead of being cared for by a loving husband, had been given over to the care of hired nurses. When Lucy eventually visited her mother, she did not find the terrifying maniac of her imagination but 'a golden-haired, blue-eyed, girlish creature, who seemed as frivolous as a butterfly, and who skipped towards us with her yellow curls decorated with natural flowers'.[22] Her mother does not know her or her father, and Lucy understands that her insanity was hereditary, a disease transmitted to her from her mother who died mad. She also finds out that her mother had been sane until she had given birth to Lucy. Following the visit to her mother in the asylum, Lady Audley says:

> I went away with the knowledge of this, and with the knowledge that the only inheritance I had to expect from my mother was – insanity!
>
> I went away with this knowledge in my mind, and with something more – a secret to keep. I was only a child of ten years old; but I felt all the weight of that burden. I was to keep the secret of my mother's madness; for it was a secret that might affect me injuriously in after-life. …[23]

Although hereditary madness was believed to have been most likely transmitted from mother to daughter, *St. Martin's Eve*,[24] a novel by Mrs Henry Wood, tells a chilling story of a woman inheriting her insanity from her mad father. Charlotte Carleton St. John murders her stepson Benja because she is jealous that he will inherit his father's title and wealth rather than her own son. Benja dies in a fire in his nursery, and Charlotte is tormented by visions of his death. The nurse who looked after Charlotte and her son, Nurse Brayford, reveals the hallucinations:

> He was always walking before her with the lighted toy, the church, the one that caused his death, you know. She had awful fits of this terror, frightening Georgy nearly to death.

When Rose Darling, Charlotte's half-sister, and Mr Frederick St. John, a relative of Charlotte's late husband, discuss her visions, they have differing interpretations of the nature of her illness: 'It must have been a sort of brain fever,' remarked Mr St. John.

'It must have been downright madness,' returned Rose. She goes on to describe Charlotte's fit of madness when she saw the lighted lanterns at the annual parade on St. Martin's Eve, 'She was quite mad when she came to fancying it was a thousand Benjas coming to torment her.'

Later, Frederick St. John thinks he detects incipient madness in Charlotte when she shows signs of being insanely jealous of Georgina Beauclerc's friendship with Sir Isaac St. John on whom she had designs, 'Frederick St. John was half frightened. If ever a woman looked mad, she looked so in that moment. Her long fingers quivered, her lips were drawn, her face was white as death.' Another evening following a further demonstration of her mad jealousy, Charlotte played the piano in such a charming manner that, 'Had all the doctors connected with Bethlehem Hospital come forward then to declare her mad, people would have laughed at them for their pains.'

The real reason for Charlotte's madness is revealed in chapter thirty-four, when the reader is informed that Charlotte's father had died mad. Mr Pym, the family doctor, tells Frederick St. John and Dean Beauclerc, 'He died raving mad, … his madness was hereditary.' In chapter thirty-six, Charlotte's insanity worsens and she has a fit of raving madness. She attacks her stepson's former nursemaid, Honour, biting, scratching and bruising her in an attack not unlike Bertha Mason's on Jane Eyre.

The concept of hereditary insanity was explained by Francis Galton, who coined the term 'Eugenics' in 1883. It encouraged 'healthy stock' to have children and discouraged the reproduction of those with mental disabilities, as madness was believed to be an inherited condition. The American gynaecologist, William Goodall (1829–1894) advocated the sterilization of the insane to try to stem the process of hereditary insanity. Although no evidence of the practice of eugenics was present in nineteenth-century mental asylum case books, the mental health of a patient's immediate relatives was recorded on their admittance. When a member of the family was known to be suffering from a similar complaint, the diagnosis given to the patient was 'hereditary insanity'.

In the real-life cases at Bethlem and other lunatic asylums, hereditary insanity was a common diagnosis. In 1856, Ann Gauntlet, a single woman aged twenty-nine, was admitted with hereditary insanity described as religious excitement. Her mother and her two brothers also suffered from mental health problems. Ann 'fancied' that she had been in France and that God had visited her in a vision: that she had been 'in the third heaven and that the Millennium had commenced'. She was very violent and her medical certificate suggested that she was a danger to herself and others. Ann believed that she was pregnant and that she was 'the woman prophesied in the Holy Scripture who, in much sorrow was to bring forth a male child'. She believed that the people around her were devils. Ann had attempted to throw herself out of the window, not much different from Bertha Mason in *Jane Eyre* throwing herself off the roof of Thornfield Hall. Bertha of course is a very complex literary character; she does not have the treatment and care that were given to Ann in Bethlem, so she ends up leaping to her death from the house she has set on fire. Ann, on the other hand, was rested, fed, treated for her constipation and was discharged from the asylum, 'recovered'. Her diagnosis of hereditary insanity and her subsequent discharge seemed to indicate that such symptoms could be spasmodic, or that hereditary insanity could be alleviated, at least on a temporary basis.

Ann Gauntlet fared a lot better than Elizabeth Eagles, a 55-year-old parasol maker who was a patient in the Hanwell Asylum in 1853. Elizabeth believed that she had 'offended the Almighty' and that she 'was about to be destroyed'. Unlike many other women, she wanted to be saved. Her cousin attributed her condition to 'her ill usage by one of her daughters who used to beat her' and when she knocked her down one time Elizabeth hurt her head so badly that she was left with a long scar on her forehead. It was also recorded that she had worked very hard but had fared badly and in consequence was 'three parts starved'. She had been in low spirits for years and had experienced some delusions. Reading everything that Elizabeth had suffered, it would seem that there were physical causes and emotional reasons for her poor mental health and probable breakdown, but the reason for her insanity was given as being 'hereditary', a diagnosis based on the fact that her mother was the result of an incestuous relationship between brother and sister, her grandparents. Her own mother was also insane. That the sins of the parents could be passed down in this way was a common belief. It was also part of evangelical doctrine that although God was 'slow to anger and abounding in steadfast love', he would, 'by no means clear the guilty, visiting the iniquity of the fathers upon the children and the children's children, to the third and the fourth generation',[25] or, in this case two generations. Elizabeth Eagles's record ended abruptly without mention of what happened to her. However, a happy outcome was hardly likely as her doctors clearly felt that she was beyond help given her lineage which was the result of incest rather than, as in the case of Ann Gauntlet, the fact that other members of her family were insane. Possibly doctors had differing opinions as to whether hereditary insanity could sometimes be assuaged by treatment; however, insanity inherited through incest would have had serious moral implications as well as clinical.

The plight of the Victorian governess

The number of governesses suffering from mental illness in asylums was a result of the problems of the nature of the job, a fact understood by Victorian female authors isolated from their own families, living in the houses of others. Loneliness was a perennial problem for these, mainly young, women and it affected their psychological and physical well-being. Charlotte Brontë said that only those who had been in the position of governess could ever understand the dark side of respectable human nature. Drawing on her own experience of loneliness when she was working as a teacher in Brussels, Brontë writes in *Villette* that:

> The world can understand the process of perishing for want of food: perhaps few persons can enter into or follow out that of going mad from solitary confinement. They see the long-buried prisoner disinterred, a maniac or an idiot![26]

Through the character of Lucy Snowe, she examines the friendless life of the governess, an educated but poor woman. Neither servant nor family, destined to be confined to the background of other people's everyday lives, underpaid, overworked and very often half-starved.

Her sister, Anne Brontë, also had first-hand knowledge of being a governess and used her experience in her novel *Agnes Grey*, which was said to be the portrayal of the torments that make up a governess's life. In narrating her own story, Anne wanted to expose the plight of many governesses to her readers. In fact, the book followed Anne's actual experience closely. Like Anne, Agnes Grey is nineteen years old, the youngest daughter of an impoverished clergyman; she comes from the North of England and has to make a living for herself because of her father's straightened circumstances. Just before Anne Brontë took up her first post as a governess, the bank failures of the 1830s impelled more middle-class women to look for paid work and the strong competition for teaching jobs meant that the governess's salary was even more depressed. The situation was so bad that in 1841 a Governesses' Benevolent Fund was founded to provide, in a delicate manner, destitute members of that class assistance in old age or illness.

The difficult life of the governess is well depicted in *Agnes Grey*. Women who chose that profession were, as we learn in *Jane Eyre,* treated with contempt by pupils such as the spoiled Blanche Ingram and her siblings; their rejection resulted in many of these women suffering from melancholia and other mental health problems. The Ingrams are depicted as being deliberately cruel and totally insensitive to the feelings of Jane Eyre who is in the room whilst they are having the following conversation about their governesses: 'Mary and I have had, I should think, a dozen at least in our day; half of them detestable and the rest ridiculous, and all incubi – were they not mama?'[27] Lady Ingram in reply to her daughter says that she has seen Jane in the room and observes, 'I noticed her: I am a judge of physiognomy, and in hers I see all the faults of her class.'

During the nineteenth century, the pseudo-science of physiognomy, or assessing a person's character from their outward appearance, gained popularity.[28] Many Victorian authors were influenced by the idea and gave detailed, physical descriptions of characters in their novels. Physiognomy claimed that a person's interiority could be read through their face; this was not a new theory, having been initially proposed by ancient Greek philosophers, discredited and then revived in the early mid-nineteenth century by Johann Kaspar Lavater, who published his work, *The Science of Physiognomy* in 1801. In studying Jane's face, Lady Ingram claims the right to comment on her character. Blanche carries on the conversation with memories of how she and her siblings made life hell for their governesses and of one, Miss Wilson, she remembers that she was not worth the trouble of vanquishing because 'Miss Wilson was a poor sickly thing, lachrymose and low spirited.'[29] Brontë has used the term 'thing' for the governess who, by the way she is described, was suffering from depression, or in nineteenth-century terminology, melancholia.

Henry Maudsley said that it was 'easy enough to recognize melancholia, as patients afflicted with it do not care to conceal their unhappiness and their delusions'.[30] Miss Wilson clearly could not hide her misery as she was tearful, but far from having delusions, her unhappiness sprang from her loneliness and the cruel way she was treated by the Ingram girls. Maudsley defined melancholia, a frequently used diagnosis for mental asylum patients, as originating in an imaginary cause. This was demonstrably not the case as many inmates had very good reason to be depressed.

'The melancholic … attributes his sufferings to some groundless extraneous cause, which either operates from without or takes possession of his body and soul, or both.'[31] Because melancholic women were seen as pale, emotional, frequently physically unwell and in low spirits the condition became linked to hysteria and therefore, as previously discussed, to their reproductive cycle. The physician George Savage concurred with this description. In 1884 he wrote that the physical symptoms of melancholia produced 'an anxious expression … the skin is generally sallow, the appetite bad, digestion imperfect, tongue moist, often tremulous and flabby, bowels confined, and general nutrition impaired'.[32] Savage states that there are both active and passive melancholia; however, what they have in common is grief and, 'Grief is a weight crushing these patients out of all their social relationships'.[33]

There was a concern amongst middle- and upper-class Victorian parents that servants, nurses and governesses could be a source of moral corruption that could affect their children. For example, nurses were suspected of masturbating baby boys to keep them from crying[34] and in so doing caused them to suffer from various mental problems in later life. In *Jane Eyre* Brontë referred to governesses as an 'anathematized race', and she hinted of something dark about that line. Lady Ingram tells Mr Rochester that she will enlighten him about their faults, not in public, but in his private ear, whilst she wags her head three times with 'portentious significancy'. Lady Ingram voices the opinion that if a governess should show signs of falling in love it demonstrates that she has an immoral tendency. When Charlotte Brontë fell in love with her teacher and employer Constantin Héger, she was punished by his wife with isolation from the family. She mirrors this treatment of the governess who dares to have romantic emotions in *Villette* in her depiction of Lucy Snowe and the love she experiences for the dark and brooding Paul Emanuel. Lucy too is ostracized by her employer Madame Beck for her presumption.

The popular perception of the Victorian governess being morally contaminated can be seen in the diagnosis given to thirty-year-old Julia Margaret East, a patient admitted to Bethlem in 1860, suspected of masturbation. Julia was a single woman from Ventor on the Isle of Wight and a governess. She was suicidal but not dangerous to others, sober, in good health and had a superior education. She was a member of the Church of England. Julia believed that she was 'cursed by God, that her relations denied her and that the food she ate was the Passover lamb with sacramental bread'. She thought that 'the shoes she wanted to wear were Jesus Christ's'. She had revelations and visions and said that she was 'possessed by the devil'. She also thought that all her relations were 'endeavouring to give her things that would kill her and that she would commit self-destruction'. Julia was given two months' leave from Bethlem so that she could go into the country, but she returned to the asylum thinner and even more restless. She was discharged, 'uncured' in May 1861. Her notes revealed that she was a woman of superior education who had spent much time abroad. Over the past few months her mind had been disordered and she had been unfit for any regular employment. She had eruptions all over her face and the catamenia were not regular which may have signalled some physical, hormonal disorder. She wandered around, was untidy in her dress and was not clean in her room nor attentive to personal cleanliness. From taking into account all the above observations it was concluded that: 'There is very little doubt that she indulges in improper practices'. This somewhat enigmatic statement would have indicated that Julia masturbated.

The Victorian governess is a familiar motif reproduced in numerous novels of the time.[35] Charlotte and Anne Brontë based their characters' experiences on first-hand knowledge. In 1839, Charlotte worked as a governess to the Sidgwick children at Stonegappe in Lothersdale. In a letter to her sister Emily on 8 June 1839, she wrote:

> I see now more clearly than I have ever done before that a private governess has no existence, it is not considered as a living and rational being except as connected with the wearisome duties that she has to fulfil.[36]

Later, on 30 June, she wrote to her friend Ellen Nussey from Swarcliffe where her employers spent the Summer at the home of Mrs Sidgwick's father.

Charlotte conceded that the countryside was beautiful but that she was unhappy in her situation:

> I will only ask you to imagine the miseries of a reserved wretch like me thrown at one into the midst of a large Family ... – when the house was filled with company – all strangers people whose faces I had never seen before – in this state of things having the charge given me of a set of pampered spoilt and turbulent children – whom I was expected constantly to amuse as well as instruct – I soon found that the constant demand on my stock of animal spirits reduced them to the lowest state of exhaustion – at times I felt and suppose seemed depressed – to my astonishment I was taken to task on the subject by Mrs. Sidgwick with a sternness of manner and a harshness of language scarcely credible – like a fool I cried most bitterly – I could not help it – my spirits quite failed me at first ... to be treated in that way merely because I was shy – and sometimes melancholy – was too bad.[37]

Novels about and first-hand accounts of the experiences of Victorian governesses and society's perception and expectations of these women[38] showed clearly why so many of them ended up in mental asylums suffering from depression and an acute sense of unworthiness.

Hysteria, eccentricity and the threat of confinement

During the nineteenth century, hysteria became a focus of both cultural and medical study. The symptoms of hysteria were so many and diverse, ranging from headaches to mania, that it frequently became the diagnosis when an illness could not be identified. The condition, seen as a particularly female ailment, was irrational, emotional and at times sexually unrestrained.[39] The physician and expert on insanity, George Man Burrows (1771–1846), wrote, 'Nervous and susceptible women between puberty and thirty years of age, and clearly the single more so than the married, are most frequently visited by hysteria.'[40] The figure of the hysterical woman became known through the work of the French neurologist Jean Martin Charcot[41] who was famous for his teaching on hysteria. He replaced the traditional ward round at the Salpêtriére Hospital in Paris with clinical demonstrations and patient interviews in the hospital amphitheatre, and his theatrical teaching caught the public imagination to the extent that hysteria became almost fashionable. From October 1885 to February

1886, Sigmund Freud attended Charcot's lectures and was so impressed that he shifted his interest from general neurology to the study of hysteria, hypnosis and other psychological issues.

The more popular medium of the novel echoed medical opinion on hysteria and authors employed it as a useful trope. Gustave Flaubert, the son of a doctor, drew the character of his heroine Emma Bovary from medical literature[42] and his novel *Madame Bovary* (1855) portrayed what was to become a typical example of female hysteria. Emma's unrealistic fantasies on life and love cause her to be dissatisfied with her dull, doctor husband. She has two hopeless love affairs and finally dies from a self-inflicted dose of arsenic, unwilling to succumb to domestic obliteration. Flaubert's description of Emma's feelings is based on the nineteenth-century, clinically accepted diagnosis of hysteria. Her suicide, whilst hysterical, would have been a plausible outcome. In England, the well-known and evocative mystery novels written by Wilkie Collins contained many of the contemporary fears around madness. He lived an unconventional, bohemian lifestyle maintaining two families yet marrying neither of his partners. He took vast quantities of opium in the form of laudanum to relieve the symptoms of ill health and was critical of the Victorian establishment. Like his friend, Charles Dickens, Collins wrote about many of the prevailing social injustices. Through his novel, *Jezebel's Daughter* (1880), he made a plea for the humane treatment of lunatics. The main protagonist of the novel is the progressive Mrs Wagner who believes that lunatics can be cured by kindness, so she removes the 'simple-minded' Jack Straw from Bethlem and takes him into her household because she feels compassion for him. 'After seeing the whip, and seeing the chains, and seeing the man – she had actually determined to commit herself to the perilous experiment which her husband would have tried, had he lived.'[43] Despite disapproval of her plan, Jack responds well, is much improved and becomes devoted to Mrs Wagner. He becomes an important character and in the end is responsible for his benefactor's recovery from an attempt to poison her.

Wilkie Collin's book *The Woman in White* published in 1860 was concerned with female insanity and false imprisonment. The story is set in the 1850s and begins with a late night encounter on Hampstead Heath between Walter Hartright, the hero, and a solitary woman dressed completely in white. The woman turns out to be Anne Catherick. Hartright helps her catch a cab;

however, a little later she meets two men who are looking for a 'woman in white', who has escaped from a lunatic asylum. The plot of the novel is sensational and complicated and revolves around the false incarceration of half-sisters, Anne Catherick and Laura Fairlie, in a mental asylum. John G. Millais, the son of the Pre-Raphaelite artist John Everett Millais, said that this first scene was based on experience. As his father and Wilkie and Charles Collins were walking one night, they met a beautiful young woman dressed in white, she hesitated, as if in distress, and then walked on. Wilkie followed her and later told his companions that she was from a good family and had fallen under the power of an unscrupulous man who had subjected her to threats and 'mesmeric influences'[44] of an alarming nature. This 'woman in white' was believed to have been Caroline Elizabeth Graves who afterwards lived with Wilkie. The novel instigated great excitement and was to prove immensely popular. It also started a franchise boom. Victorians could buy *Woman in White* perfume, cloaks and bonnets. It was said that Thackeray sat up all night reading it and it was admired by Prince Albert. Critics argue that *The Woman in White* was particularly relevant to certain disturbing aspects of mid-nineteenth century life so making it especially sensational for the contemporary reader.

Charles Dickens, despite the fact that he was a keen supporter of asylum reform, colluded with John Forster, the secretary to the Lunacy Commission, and John Connolly, the renowned mad doctor, to gain a separation from his wife Catherine. In 1858, he charged her with mental illness and alluded to the possibility of her confinement in a lunatic asylum.[45] He traced her disorder to her supposed maternal difficulties in 1850–1851, referring to her reputed bout of post-natal depression following the birth of a sickly ninth child, Dora, in 1850. Although her daughter made an apparent recovery in February 1951, she died suddenly in April. Catherine's ensuing 'breakdown' was a normal reaction to the loss of her child. In 1857, Dickens met and fell in love with the young actress Ellen Ternan. He was forty-five and she eighteen. They began a secret affair which came to light in 1858 when Catherine opened a packet containing a gold bracelet, a gift for Ellen from her husband. Catherine and Charles separated that year after twenty-two years of marriage. The threat of incarcerating his wife in a mental asylum was used to hasten their estrangement.

Reports of cases of false incarceration in lunatic asylums were used by the penny press to whip up the imagination of the general reader. Just before and during the serialization of *The Woman in White* in the popular magazine *All the Year Round,* which was edited by Charles Dickens, a select committee of the House of Commons was set up to investigate the care and treatment of lunatics and their property. Whilst stating that the County Asylums were, on the whole, satisfactory, the committee considered the call for the abolition of private asylums. It came to the conclusion that even though several of the houses, both in the metropolis and the country, were not fit for purpose, this would not be possible. However, taking into consideration the pecuniary advantage to the owners of private asylums in accepting patients, there should be some regulation concerning certification of madness. The committee also concluded that the recommendation of the Commissioners of Lunacy, that it should be 'made compulsory upon the friends of all the patients to visit them, or delegate someone to visit them periodically and ascertain by personal inspection the accommodation and comforts provided for them', deserved 'consideration'. The final conclusion arrived at by the committee went against the widespread perceptions of the times:

> We do not for one moment underrate the importance of protecting the lunatic as much as may be practicable from unjust confinement or improper treatment … Had the evidence even shown that the popular belief in the too frequently unjust detention and improper treatment of the insane had been to some extent correct – a belief which, by the way gave rise to this inquiry, but which the evidence clearly showed to be almost entirely without foundation, in so far as asylums were concerned –.[46]

Woman in White was obviously echoing contemporary fears expressed in the non-fictional stories of women in asylums at this time.

Patients frequently believed that they were being poisoned, usually by members of their family, abducted and assaulted. Susannah Foot was in the City of London Mental Asylum in 1866 said to be suffering from 'delusional insanity'. She believed that 'the Prince of Wales was her husband and that she had chloroform administered to her every night'. Whilst she was under the influence of the chloroform she thought she was criminally assaulted by three men. She also believed that she has had 'a model taken of her nude body and that she was pregnant'. Patients in asylums either consciously or unconsciously reflected contemporary fears when expressing their delusions. By the 1850s chloroform was regularly used as an anaesthetic and was being produced on a commercial basis. It was the subject of much debate especially when it was known that Queen Victoria had allowed its use when she gave birth to her eighth child Prince Leopold. Chloroform was reported as being used as a tool for muggers and abductors as witnessed by a letter to *The Times* in September 1850 in which the writer said that he was robbed in Regent's Park by two young men who rendered him insensible by placing a chloroform-soaked mask over his face. A sensation novel like *The Woman in White* could induce all sorts of fears around mental health and abduction and it could, and did, also mirror fact. The concerns that men were in the habit of having their wives or unruly members of their family falsely locked up in an asylum on the say so of just two doctors were strong at this time and not a short-lived phenomenon.[47] Fifteen years later in 1875, Mrs George Weldon accused her husband of attempting to sell her house and put her into a lunatic asylum. She even self-published a book about her experiences: *How I Escaped the Mad Doctors: A Thrilling Narrative of Personal Experience, Showing by What Means Large Numbers of Perfectly Sane and Intellectually Endowed Individuals of Both Sexes Are Immured in Madhouses for Life, at the Instigation of Relatives; in Carrying out Whose Behests a Class of Men Derive a Lucrative Trade. An Appeal to Every Noble-Hearted Englishman and Englishwoman to Cry Aloud for the Reform of the Lunacy Laws.* In these few words she summed up Victorian fears concerning the destination of so-called lunatics.

Victorian novelists frequently attributed the inspiration for certain characters in their books to people they encountered in their everyday life, for example, Wilkie Collin's inspiration for his woman in white. The streets of nineteenth-century London in particular afforded plenty of scope through the eccentric behaviour of some of the citizens. As seen in Chapter 2, Elizabeth James, an eccentric, London character who became a patient in Bethlem in 1821 was one such woman who could have easily become a Dickens or Collins character.[48] Miss Havisham from *Great Expectations* was supposed to have been based on a woman whom Charles Dickens, as a boy, saw wandering in Berners and Oxford Street. She was always dressed in white and was rumoured to have become mad due to her rejection by a wealthy Quaker. Miss Havisham is presented as suffering from what John Conolly classified as 'hysterical insanity'[49]; however, her illness was incomprehensible to most Victorian readers who found it difficult to differentiate between eccentricity and madness. Eccentric characters were more of a common sight in nineteenth-century society than they are today. The asylum records show many such people but they were usually only admitted when their behaviour became too anti-social to be tolerated by those around them.

Madness and the weaker sex

A general discourse of the infantilization of women with their accompanying emotional and sexual instability was found in much nineteenth-century writing; for example, the mentally afflicted Anne Catherick in *The Woman in White* is seen as infantile. Well-bred young ladies and adult women were supposed to be innocent and childlike; they even had the same legal status as children in Victorian England, as non-competent dependents. On marriage, a woman's legal rights and obligations were absorbed by those of her husband, she was not allowed the vote and she lacked the possibility of higher education. Powerful stereotypes of femininity which portrayed the innocent, childlike woman were disseminated throughout society through religion, law and education, reinforcing the subservient role of women. These images continued to exert a powerful hold on the Victorian literary imagination; however, the representation of the girlish woman was not confined to male authors, even female authors were apt to present their protagonists as weak, feeble and childlike, unwittingly influenced by the stereotypes around them. In *Jane Eyre*, Charlotte Brontë recognized the problem of the stifled woman:

> Women are supposed to be very calm generally: but women feel just as men feel; they need exercise for their faculties, and a field for their efforts as much as their brothers do; they suffer from too rigid a restraint, too absolute a stagnation, precisely as men would suffer; and it is narrow-minded in their more privileged fellow-creature to say that they ought to confine themselves to making puddings and knitting stockings, to playing on the piano and embroidering bags. It is thoughtless to condemn them, or laugh at them, if they seek to do more or learn more than custom has pronounced necessary for their sex.[50]

Yet, later in the novel she has Jane describing herself as 'little' and Mr Rochester referring to her as 'a wild, frantic bird that is rending its own plumage in its desperation,'[51] and 'you strange – you almost unearthly thing! … You – poor and obscure, and small and plain as you are … ' Emphasizing Jane's childlike stature and uncontrolled passion. Even Brontë, who was aware of women's enforced, submissive role in society, echoes the sentiments of male authors.

In *Lady Audley's Secret*, Mary Elizabeth Braddon describes Lady Audley, newly married to her 'generous baronet', as 'happy as a child surrounded by new and costly toys'. Her step-daughter, Miss Alicia, showed 'undisguised contempt for her step-mother's childishness and frivolity' however:

> Lucy was better loved and more admired than the baronet's daughter. That very childishness had a charm which few could resist. The innocence and candour of an infant beamed in Lady Audley's fair face, and shone out of her large and liquid blue eyes. The rosy lips, the delicate nose, the profusion of fair ringlets, all contributed to preserve to her beauty the character of extreme youth and freshness. … her fragile figure, which she loved to dress in heavy velvets and stiff rustling silks, till she looked like a child tricked out for a masquerade, was as girlish as if she had just left the nursery.[52]

Braddon goes on to describe Lady Audley's amusements as being childish. She did not care for reading or study of any kind, but preferred playing with her jewellery and gifts. It is her infantile qualities that make her uniquely attractive to men. It is also a veiled warning of what lies behind her presumed innocence.

The infantilization of women had its roots in some pseudo-scientific theories such as the one put forward by the Rev. John Jessop wrote in his book, *Woman* (1851):

> Moreover, the humbler sphere we assign to woman is precisely that for which her whole constitution is predisposed and as it were, instinctively adapted. Her more slender and fragile build, her more rapid beating of the pulses, her more lively sensibility of nerve, her greater delicacy of organization and of feature, all contribute to constitute her the 'weaker vessel'.[53]

Jessop, of course, blurred the medical facts to ideological ends. A woman's pulse rate is not determined by her gender, but by her physical fitness, as is a man's. A child, however, does have a more rapid pulse than an adult, so in this instance the woman was being imbued with childlike qualities. Because women were perceived as being weaker than men, both intellectually and physically, it followed that they were more prone to mental illnesses, as was demonstrated in the character of Lady Audley.

The curse of poverty

Class, like gender, was an important consideration in the treatment of madness. Poverty was certainly fear provoking in Victorian England especially if you were insane. Although conditions improved greatly when the county asylums came into being in 1845, patients, often referred to as pauper lunatics, who would have previously been sent to the workhouse or an uninspected private madhouse did not usually fare as well as those from a higher class. The rich could avoid the stigma of certification by keeping mad relatives at home or by seeking private care. For a large fee, the affluent lunatic might lodge privately with a doctor or be sent to one of the large private asylums such as Laverstock or Ticehurst that catered to the wealthy. Another option was to ship the patient off to the continent to be hidden away in a maison de santé. In literature, Miss Havisham, in *Great Expectations*, is saved from incarceration in a lunatic asylum by her wealth. Instead, Satis House becomes her prison where she confines herself, apart from society, because she has failed as a Victorian woman. The affluent Mr Rochester in *Jane Eyre* chooses to keep his lunatic wife at home under the care of Grace Poole who had been an attendant in an asylum, whereas Lady Audley, in *Lady Audley's Secret,* is dispatched to Belgium, much to her horror:

> Sir Michael Audley's wicked wife laid her hand suddenly upon Robert's arm, and pointed with the other hand to this curtained window. "I know where you have brought me," she said. "This is a MAD-HOUSE." … "What is this place Robert Audley?" she cried fiercely. "Do you think I am a baby, that you may juggle with and deceive me – what is it? It is what I said just now is it not?"
>
> "It is a maison de santé, my lady," the young man answered gravely.
>
> "A maison de santé," she repeated. "Yes they manage these things better in France. In England we should call it a madhouse."[54]

Lady Audley is told to repent and at this point in the novel Braddon says that she hated herself and hated her own beauty, even the French doctor refers to her as a 'beautiful devil'. She says to Robert Audley:

> I would laugh at you and defy you if I dared. ... I would kill myself and defy you if I dared. But I am a poor, pitiful coward and have been so from the first. Afraid of my mother's horrible inheritance; afraid of poverty: afraid of George Talboys; afraid of you.[55]

In this utterance, Lady Audley articulates fears around madness. Poverty, heredity, suicide and powerlessness.

By the 1870s countless inmates were 'warehoused' in the big county asylums and in many cases forgotten about. In this aspect working-class women frequently suffered the same fate of being 'buried' or lost to the world as their better off sisters. In March 1871, 38-year-old Frances Mercy Adenham was admitted to Colney Hatch from the workhouse. Frances was unmarried and her mania was said to have been caused by 'disappointment in marriage'. She spent nineteen years in Colney Hatch before being discharged aged fifty-seven. Thirty-two-year-old Mary Stinson, a single servant was also sent to Colney Hatch from the workhouse in 1871. She had experienced the onset of 'mania', following the death of an illegitimate child. She spent six years in Colney Hatch before being discharged, 'relieved' in 1877. Other women such as Elizabeth Hodges, a 24-year-old single domestic servant, spent nine years in the asylum suffering from 'melancholia' brought on by 'disappointment in love', and 'sunstroke', an unusual medical diagnosis. Over-exposure to hot sun could be attributed to a patient who had been overseas, but Elizabeth had presumably not been out of England. Sophia Gaylord, a single servant, was incarcerated for ten years following 'an attack of mania' brought about by 'a love affair'. Martha Lloyd, a nineteen-year-old, single match box maker from Bethnal Green, suffered from 'melancholia following abandonment by her lover'. She was admitted to Colney Hatch in good health in November 1872 but died in June 1874. Matchbox making was well known as being sweated labour carried out by women and young girls in the East End of London, particularly Bethnal Green. Martha Lloyd would have been on the bottom rung of society and one of the poorest.

The forgotten inmates of the Victorian asylums reflected the very real fear of being diagnosed as mad and then lost to the world. The social problems of the age, including poverty, unemployment and child mortality, were believed to be amongst the causes of insanity as were religious mania, hysteria and heredity. Nineteenth-century novelists harnessed these anxieties in order to make their novels both sensational and realistic. In *The Lazy Tour of Two Idle Apprentices*[56] Charles Dickens has Mr Francis Goodchild describe his visit to a lunatic asylum. He says that he observed 'the usual thing', which was:

> Long groves of blighted men-and-women-trees; interminable avenues of hopeless faces; numbers, without the slightest power of really combining for any earthly purpose; a society of human creatures who have nothing in common but they have lost all the power of being humanly social with one another.[57]

Such a gloomy picture must have struck the readers of *Household Words*, the weekly magazine edited by Charles Dickens in the 1850s, as depressing and hopeless, a fate to be avoided at all costs.

Male Asylum Patients

Lost souls of every type were there: and yet
The hell of one was not another's hell.
Nor needed separate prisons to adjust
The righteous meed of punishment to each.
As they had sinn'd, they suffer'd.[1]

Edward Henry Bickersteth, *Yesterday, Today and Forever*

Victorian, middle-class masculinity can be summed up as an ideology of spirituality and earnestness, which was displayed in men's moral courage, athleticism and stoicism.[2] Men were seen as unemotional and more rational than women. A married man was head of the household, the 'pater familias', and ruled those within it; however, it was also his duty to protect his wife and family. Marriage was considered good for men; it gave them an outlet for their sexual passions and safeguarded their mental health. W.A.F. Browne (1805–1985), medical superintendent of the Montrose Lunatic Asylum, said in 1837 on the subject of marriage:

> To man it is the shield against himself and his passions; he seeks and finds in it joy, solace, and support … it prevents the mind from retiring on itself, acts as a barrier against hidden sorrows, gives employment to out noblest qualities and … because it yields no strong or permanent excitement, it is an antidote to insanity.[3]

As the century developed, the virtues of a healthy body as well as a healthy mind became important. For middle- and upper-class men, athleticism was nurtured in the public schools which were exclusively male establishments. Men were discouraged from showing their feelings and the British 'stiff upper lip' was required from boys as well as their fathers. The repression of emotions was also seen as the mark of a real man and over-indulgence was considered weak and unmanly. Browne added, 'A large proportion of the physical causes and influence of ambition, speculation and dissipation are confined in their operation to men.'[4] In other words, men should observe moderation in all things in order to protect themselves from madness.

It is this view of nineteenth-century masculinity that has passed into popular history; however, it was different for the working-class man. The 'respectable' artisan or labouring man would have formed his identity in his employment. To a certain extent, he mirrored his upper- and middle-class peers in adherence to religion and family, and of course there were the good, hard-working, God-fearing men who aimed to follow the principles of decent, manly conduct.[5] Nevertheless, working-class men were perceived to be in less control of their emotions than the better educated; nearer to animals in their irrational and sometimes 'beastly' behaviour. A train of thought held that they were more inclined to violence. The Victorian psychiatrist Dr Thomas Monro (1759–1833) stated that under his superintendence, 'gentlemen' were never chained but that such measures were necessary for the poor in public establishments. This observation was considered an error of judgement by Browne, but appears to have been a popular perception, fuelled by contemporary writers of fiction such as Arthur Morrison, author of books set in London, East End slums.

In his novel, *A Child of the Jago* (1896), Morrison describes a family, the Ropers, who move into the Jago, an East End slum and are despised by their neighbours because of their attempts to be respectable. He describes them as 'interlopers'; the father, a pale cabinet maker, was out of work and so the family had fallen on 'evil times'. His wife is disliked because of her 'neatly kept clothes, her exceeding use of soap and water, her aloofness from gossip'. Mr Roper was particularly disapproved of because he 'did not drink or brawl, nor beat his wife, nor do anything all day but look for work'.[6] Although *A Child of The Jago* is a work of fiction, Morrison was born in Poplar and spent his youth in the East End of London, so he had first-hand experience of lower-class masculinity and would have been aware that drink was an important element in working-class lives. It symbolized manliness and adulthood, and spending money on drink was the prerogative of the working man. It was also linked with problems in holding down a job, domestic violence and insanity. The main, moral reasons for male admissions into the Colney Hatch asylum in 1864 were intemperance and debauchery.

Whatever their class, men held the power in Victorian England. There was a system of male supremacy, authority and sex privilege which was a social construction and meant that women from all levels of society were subordinated and controlled. This structure of patriarchal privilege was upheld by men and demanded a certain type of masculine behaviour to sustain it. Middle- and upper-class men held the moral high ground and dominated educated opinion, whereas working-class men were to be of a lower order, more aggressive and unreasonable.

Mid-nineteenth-century male patients

Specific ideas about the madness of men and women abounded at this time. Dr J.G. Millingen asserted:

> Their (women) delirium is chiefly religious or erotic, complicated with hysteria, and pride in the frequent attendant on the malady which it had ushered in. Female lunatics are in general more deceitful and dangerous than men. Men are more subject to maniacal violence and more easily cured, and less subject to relapses.[7]

Such a gendered statement can be analysed in comparing a sample of male case notes from the inmates of Bethlem, Colney Hatch and Hanwell asylums in the second half of the nineteenth century to those of women. J.G. Millingen's belief that men were more subject to maniacal violence was borne out by their asylum records. In making a comparison with the female records, a marked difference in how their various diagnoses were arrived at became obvious. Even when the man had been admitted for the same or similar reason as that of the woman, the way the illness was manifested was different in each gender. For example, Josiah Smith, a 27-year-old, single errand boy from Clerkenwell, was admitted to Bethlem in January 1855, suffering from depression. He was not suicidal but dangerous to others. Josiah was incoherent and said that he had been 'possessed by the devil' to whom he had sold himself. He supposed himself to be 'occupied by evil spirits'. He was violent and dangerous to those around him especially his mother who he had 'attempted to kill with a poker'. The patient was described as being 'very thin and pale with an unhealthy expression'. His health was bad and he was very deformed by a 'lateral curvature of the spine'. Josiah was extremely depressed and rarely spoke, even when he was asked a question; he was peevish, fretful, bad tempered and obstinate. He was 'disposed to refuse his food'. This moderately educated young man had a depressive illness, which, like many females, he expressed through the medium of religion. However, far from feeling that he was doomed because of his sin and unworthiness, he believed that he had sold his soul to Satan and his possession by evil made him attack his mother. Luckily for Josiah, who was clearly physically unwell, his cure was brought about chiefly by food, rest and calm and he was discharged in April 1856. Life for a poor errand boy was hard in Victorian England. Josiah's life would have been a fight for survival especially as he was physically deformed. It would seem that Bethlem's enlightened regime of nourishment and relaxation was enough to raise his spirits and calm his violence.

In the same year, the day after Josiah Smith entered Bethlem, 36-year-old John Meears, married with a child of five weeks, joined him. His condition was diagnosed as the result of 'failure in business', having been unsuccessful as a publican before becoming a coachman to a noble family. He was not suicidal, but violent. He told the doctor that he had 'personal communication with The Almighty and that two angels were in attendance upon him'. The doctor, Edward William Eton from Windsor, said that he had witnessed John stripping himself naked whenever he was left alone, apparently without any objective. He persisted in lying in bed and spent an unusual time in the water closet saying that God had ordered him to stay there. He was worried about being sent to an asylum. Although he appeared to have improved in both his physical and mental health, the doctor believed, from John's peculiar look and behaviour, that he was still 'subject to spectral illusions and unquestionably insane'. The second certifying doctor added that John 'fancied that a host of devils were outside his window' and would not have the curtains drawn. He lacked expression because he had partial paralysis of the face: 'there is very little doubt that incipient paralysis is the form of insanity in this case'. In the 1880s, incipient paralysis was linked to syphilis as it was known to travel to the brain and cause physical weakness, grandiose delusions and sometimes violent behaviour. If this was John's underlying problem, it would have explained his conduct. However, whatever the medical or psychological reason, his violence and ostentatious, religious fantasies were particularly male. He was discharged 'uncured' eight months later.

Men with religious delusions were far more likely than their female counterparts to believe that they had supernatural powers or that they were a deity. These delusions often made them physically dangerous. Thirty-year-old William Bull, a single, sober labourer from Shotteswell in Warwickshire, was dangerous, but not suicidal, when he was admitted to Bethlem in March 1885. He said that he was Jesus Christ and he 'went to heaven twice last night and returned to Shotteswell'. He believed that all the world was his private property, that the Devil visited him and they had long conversations. Dr Henry Shorthouse of Banbury noted his 'impious assertion that he was the Saviour of mankind' and pronounced him simpleminded and only fit for manual work. Within six months, William was 'cured' and discharged from the asylum. Samuel Denton, another patient in Bethlem, was not 'simple minded' like William, but a young medical assistant from Sussex who had received a superior education. He was also recorded as dangerous but not suicidal. Samuel saw himself as a prophet and able to perform miracles. Unfortunately, the miracle he planned to execute was that of turning all his relatives into dogs. He was also under the impression that London was the Babylon foretold in the Bible, there would be 'an end of time in ten years' and 'the Queen was a woman of immoral and dissolute habits whilst the Emperor of Russia was a paragon of perfection who would eventually triumph over the world'. It was strange that Samuel's opinions on London, which were fairly common at this time, should have been recorded as evidence of his insanity. His views on the Queen and the Emperor might have been 'unusual' in Victorian England, but surely not a symptom of madness. Possibly he was seen as being politically dangerous as well as a potential threat to his family and his symptoms of insanity lay in his belief that he was a powerful prophet who, at the age of twenty-five, could change the world around him and foretell the future.

Even when men sank into despondency and despair and explained their feelings through religious language, they were seen as having a solid, material reason for their depression. It was not put down to any gender-specific, physical cause, as was usually the case with women. When Joseph Hall suffered his second attack of religious mania at the age of forty-nine, he was put into the asylum and said to be suffering from 'anxiety in business'. He was a solicitor with seven children and was experiencing religious delusions. Joseph believed that his soul was lost and that he 'had a hell within him'. He refused to eat and often raved at and called upon the Almighty. He prayed a lot, hardly ever slept and was extremely constipated. Dr Thomas Remington of Brixton saw Joseph as in: 'a state of mental despondency due to his failure as a solicitor. He is struggling for a livelihood.' Luckily for Joseph he was able to rest and be fed well in Bethlem. He relieved his bowels and after four months of care he was discharged 'cured'.

In her book *Shattered Nerves*, Janet Oppenheim has pointed out that anxiety and worry about work were dangerously close to what was considered to be a feminine condition. Men were seen to generate their own mental breakdown, usually through some sort of failure, whereas women were perceived to have very little personal control over their psychological well-being.[8] Joseph's failure as a solicitor and worry about feeding his large family were a perfectly respectable, manly reason for falling prey to religious mania. As previously noted, a prerequisite of Victorian masculinity was a man's ability to provide and care for his household.

Another middle-class man who appeared to be suffering from a serious mental breakdown was moved from Peckham House, an asylum that had a reputation for being brutal and cruel, to Bethlem in August 1858. Twenty-eight-year-old George Sprately, married with four children, was a stockbroker. He became 'incoherent in conversation' and 'violent and destructive of things in general'; for example, he would tear his clothes. He showed symptoms of madness in his general behaviour, lying on the floor rolling over and over, kicking and knocking himself and talking to imaginary beings, sometimes in a loud voice. He was 'dirty in his habits', an expression which usually meant that he masturbated, and destructive, frequently refusing his food whilst at other times eating and drinking 'inordinately'. George had committed acts of violence previous to his admission requiring several men to restrain him; he had also had to be 'bound down' by his father in law. The instigation for this extraordinary behaviour and inner turmoil was given as 'change of fortune'; his violence appears to be accepted as a masculine response to his 'difficulties in pecuniary matters' which was said to be the cause of his insanity. Unfortunately for George, even though his diagnosis would have protected his masculinity, he could not be cured and was discharged from Bethlem after a year. Whether he went home to be cared for by his wife, returned to Peckham House or had to go to the workhouse was not recorded.

Of course not all male asylum patients were violent or had grandiose delusions nor were they always the victims of anxiety over work and money. Some suffered from paranoia. Thomas William Wilson, an independent minister of superior education and good bodily health, who, despite all his advantages in life and a wife and five children, had, by the age of fifty, sunk into a 'slough of despond' and become very suicidal. Like many women of a similar age, Thomas believed that he had committed, what his wife referred to as, 'the most vile crimes' of which she was certain that he had never been guilty. However, had that sin been a secret, adultery for example, she might have been ignorant of his wrongdoing. There was no suggestion that his melancholic state could have been due to his age or gender as would be the norm in a comparable case of a female; and although he believed that he was damned because of his sins, he was more violent in his delusions than most women. He used words such as 'outlawed' and believed that his wife and family would suffer all kinds of 'indignities and ill usage'. The belief that personal sin would cause suffering to others was not an exclusively male fear, but as the 'pater familias' and a clergyman, Thomas would have felt his responsibility towards his wife and family keenly. Because he believed he had no hope of forgiveness in this world or the next, he had attempted suicide and had implored other people to kill him. It was clear from Thomas's second certificate of insanity that he was prey to paranoia. The doctor reported that the day he saw him he was convinced that he was being watched and would be stripped and pelted by the mob and even torn to pieces. He was also convinced that he was being pursued by the police. Whilst in Bethlem (1858) Thomas was said to be in an extreme state of melancholy, so depressed that he attempted to hang himself by tying his handkerchief to the asylum gas pipe, but there was no opinion given as to why he was so mentally ill. Thomas did not go home cured but simply transferred to an asylum in Norwich where presumably he became a long-term patient, something that was not allowed in Bethlem.

Private asylums

The experiences of men in private lunatic asylums seem to have been varied and, according to some sources, often depended on how much money they had to bribe the keepers and owners. Apart from a few well-run and well-documented private mental hospitals, such as Ticehurst and the York Retreat, records of the smaller establishments have been destroyed. However, Victorian writers recounted stories about what was perceived to go on within their walls. Charles Dickens was aware of the reputation of these places as, in his novel *David Copperfield*, he tells the reader that David's aunt, Betsy Trotwood had rescued the simpleminded Mr Dick from a private asylum where he was being mistreated. He also serialized Charles Reade's novel *Very Hard Cash* (later *Hard Cash*) in his journal, *All the Year Round* in 1863. The story of a sane, young man, Alfred Hardie, being imprisoned in a private lunatic asylum by his wicked father caused concern amongst its readers because of its attack on private asylums.

The Victorian journalist John Mitford maintained that private madhouse owners would take anybody for their own financial gain. Prefaced by an angry tirade against Thomas Warburton,[9] Mitford listed some of the inmates of his asylum, Whitmore House, who should not be there.[10] Men such as the brother of the radical, political reformer Mr Henry 'orator' Hunt.[11] Hunt's brother was, in Mitford's opinion, more of a fool than a lunatic. In the asylum he was treated like a dog, cleaned the boots and the shoes of the keepers and performed other menial household tasks for which he was generally beaten for his pains. The reason given for the harsh treatment of this unfortunate man was that his brother Henry owed Warburton £700 in fees. Mitford did not know if this was true or not but believed that Mr Henry Hunt would be better employed denouncing such 'receptacles' as Hoxton House than using his eloquence on behalf of other causes. In another, different, reference to money, Mitford wrote about a Mr Church whom he said was not mad, but very wealthy:

> He had done the Grand Tour and had brought home all the foreign vices that degrade most of our continental travellers. … He was in the habit of committing a foul offence for which the law assigns the punishment of death and would have been very justly hanged; but Mr. Warburton's house received him as a lunatic and saved his neck.[12]

In nineteenth-century England, sodomy, or what Mitford referred to as 'a foul offence' was illegal and until 1861, was allegedly punishable by hanging. Mr Church was not incarcerated in the asylum because his sexual misdeeds were a symptom or causes of madness, but to protect him from the law, and, far from trying to stop Mr Church carrying on with his sexual misconduct, Warburton was said to have repeatedly committed the same 'crime' with him in a room at the end of the house. Mitford was scandalized that this man, the son of a colonel, was allowed to behave like a 'depraved monster' and then sat in the parlour with the other patients both male and female as though nothing had happened. The only reason that his 'enormities' were looked on as a matter of course was because he distributed his money amongst the keepers. In other words, he was bribing them in exchange for their silence

Religious excitement

Marked differences existed between the reasons for the incarceration of men and women in mental hospitals, noticeable in the cases of 'Religious Mania' or where religion was cited as the catalyst for or 'exciting' the patient's condition. Gender has been highlighted previously in the language used in the defining and diagnosis of madness depending on the sex of the sufferer. However, madwomen used religious language to express their sadness and despair in a way not usual in their fellow, male patients, as a sample of men's case books can show.

In the male patient records of Bethlem Hospital from the mid-1850s, the reasons given for 'excitement' varied from over-study, excitement about going to America to a cold, fright, intemperance, disappointed affection or many variations on business troubles. One man was said to have gone insane because of the Indian climate, another because he had consulted a great many quack doctors, some of whom had told him that he was suffering with spermatorrhoea and that his 'brain was passing off with his urine'. Spermatorrhoea[13] was a condition of excessive, involuntary discharge of semen. It was considered a form of sexual dysfunction and was associated with masturbation. Men's vital life force and energy were thought to be connected to their sperm. However, the men whose insanity was said to have been 'excited' by religion were generally diagnosed as suffering from delusions caused by over-study of the Bible or an unhealthy interest in religious matters.

In Colney Hatch and Hanwell asylums, male patients were diagnosed with religious delusions, but they were generally more violent than those in Bethlem.

Epilepsy, dementia, masturbation and general paralysis were the main reasons given for their madness, along with intemperance, poverty and heredity. Some men were seen to have gone mad due to an accident, particularly when they had suffered a blow to the head. What they had in common was that their delusions were self-aggrandising and mainly to do with money and position. They used God and Satan to make themselves more important and to threaten people, as in the case of William Lay, a sixty-year-old Baptist butcher who was admitted to Colney Hatch in 1855; he called himself an 'angel of light' and believed that nobody could kill him. His mental illness was recorded as being caused by poverty, which was a fairly common diagnosis at this time. 'Adverse circumstances', 'including business anxieties' and 'pecuniary difficulties', were recognized by psychiatrists as stimulating mental health problems and even causing total breakdown resulting in general paralysis. Commenting on the above, George Savage wrote:

> This variety of cause acts mostly on men, while domestic trouble, etc., falls most heavily on women. This cause also rarely acts suddenly, but is long preparing for the disaster by petty worries, anxieties, loss in position and social regard, which may be often followed later by penury, starvation, or over-stimulation induced by anxiety and sleeplessness ... Every year patients are admitted who have sustained severe money losses.[14]

It is probable that William's butchery business had failed, plunging him into despair over the distress this would have caused him and his family. At sixty years old he could have been anticipating a harsh future, possibly in the workhouse.

More violent was Thomas Streeter, a 44-year-old confectioner, a member of the Church of England, who was diagnosed with religious mania in 1862. He said that he knew Christ, had seen him frequently and believed that he too had been crucified and was now 'The Prince of Peace'. However, far from being peaceful, he went around the neighbourhood raving that he was Christ crucified and his wife, who he attempted to murder, was a doomed woman. He also tried to kill the vicar. No reason was given for Thomas's condition and no change in his behaviour was mentioned until he died, following a severe bout of diarrhoea, four years after his admittance. Another violent confectioner was 36-year-old John Keogh from Oxford Street who was married with two children. He had an attack of insanity which lasted for four days and resulted in his incarceration in Bethlem in January 1857. Although he was well educated and originally believed to be of sober habits, he suddenly became 'anxious, suicidal and dangerous to others'. He 'swore furiously', spat in people's faces and 'vowed to do violence to himself and his wife'. His 'ravings and incessant talking' were first about religion, followed by profanities. Keogh believed that everyone about him wished to do him injury. His delusion was recorded as being religious, believing that he had a mission from God to convert all sinners. He gave the cause of his illness as his suffering from a cold and fever and, thinking that 'the doctor could do him no good', he self-medicated with large quantities of port wine, which made him completely disorientated. When the intoxication passed off however, the symptoms of insanity remained. Records show what treatment was given to Keogh to alleviate his suffering. He was given morphia and warm baths, but these did little to help him. He was then given castor oil to cure his constipation and his case notes register that since his bowels had been 'freely acted on', the symptoms had 'much abated'[15] and he was comparatively calm; however, this depended on the effect of the morphia. Several days later the doctors undertook a new trial with medicine but Keogh's condition worsened. When he was allowed to attend the Sunday service in the hospital chapel, he became 'excited and abusive' because he was not allowed to stay and take the sacrament. Nothing more about his treatment was noted, save that after nearly two months in Bethlem he was sent home 'on trial' for a month after which he returned to the asylum and was discharged, 'cured'.

The effects of alcohol and general paralysis

In the case of John Keogh, the patient admitted to having drunk 'large quantities of port wine', which made him disorientated; however, when the intoxication wore off, he was still insane. Strong drink and intemperance were common instigators of madness according to male patient case books and alcohol was identified as causing various forms of mental disorder, including excitability, depression, dementia and stupor often resulting in paralysis. Chronic insanity, or the 'insanity of alcoholization', had symptoms, including: 'hallucinations of hearing, and sometimes of touch, leading to the belief in persecution by spies, mesmeric action, magnetic influence, and like evil agencies; the memory is usually much enfeebled, the intellect dull, and the higher sentiments are blunted.[16] When men with an alcohol problem were placed into an asylum, they had to abstain from drinking and the withdrawal symptoms, delirium tremens, could cause hallucinations and physical problems such as a high fever. Dr Andrew Wynter (1819–1876), a Victorian specialist in insanity, wrote:

> In the hallucinations that occur in those suffering from delirium tremens, as a rule the visions are in the form of animals running about the room or over the bed, making grimaces … Persons will appear to follow patients affected in this way, who immediately disappear when any attempt is made to clutch them. Any chance object seems to give rise to hallucinations in this disease.[17]

Another danger of strong drink could be observed in the effect it had on the unborn child: 'The temperance and teetotal folks are not aware of the powerful weapon they have in their hands in the known fact that persistent drunkards, in nine cases out of ten, plant the seeds of insanity and the allied nervous diseases in their offspring.'[18]

In this assertion, Wynter speaks of drunken parents so he is putting the blame onto the fathers as well as the mothers; this is because he believes in the moral effects of drunkenness on children. 'In the persistent use of alcohol we trace, without the smallest doubt, the planting of the germs of mental as well as bodily disease in the blood, and we do not doubt that it is the cause of a very large percentage of the lunacy in the country.'[19] As drunkenness was seen as a 'moral' affliction and one that could be avoided, it was not surprising that it was linked with sin and guilt in the minds of the sufferers. These feelings were reinforced by the religious teaching of the day, especially the supporters of the temperance movement which advocated abstention from alcoholic beverages.

Alcoholism produced 'every shade of mental symptom which may be seen more permanently in general paralysis',[20] a disease that had, by the mid-nineteenth century, become linked to syphilis and was a common diagnosis for men. General paralysis was recognized by ideas of power and grandeur found in the sufferers before they deteriorated into dementia. The connection between these exalted delusions with religion was fairly common in the male patients studied.[21] One such case was James Bentley, a 31-year-old butler from Tooting, South London. Bentley was a single man of sober habits with a moderate education, who was admitted to Bethlem in March 1857. He believed that reading religious books had given him 'direct influence over the sun so that he could control its shining'. His other delusions included imagining that people were talking to him and urging him to do things that he would not otherwise have done, believing that people were 'speaking to him from his bowels' and that rats and mice were intentionally placed around him to 'annoy' him. He became violent and attempted to jump out of the window, being urged, as he said, by 'persons calling him'. There was a slow onset of insanity and further, grandiose fantasies. He said that he was King James the first and that he had supernatural powers over the heavenly bodies. James had the symptoms of general paralysis of the insane, and yet he was diagnosed as suffering from religious mania.

Victorian men in business

By the middle of the nineteenth century men's masculinity became deeply imbedded in what they did for a living.[22] Men pursued commercial interests and trades were increasing in numbers and variation, largely due to the improvement of transport. Because of the importance of their occupation, not only to the maintenance of home and family, but also to their feelings of self-esteem, men could, and did, turn to religion when their commercial endeavours failed and they needed to find some explanation for their misfortune. Unfortunately, this could lead them into mad and delusional behaviour.

Class was important to the Victorians and the working classes were divided between the labouring class, the artisan and the more educated working man. Like their middle-class counterparts, work was largely what defined them but unlike those who had supportive families, savings or a profession, when they lost their job, for whatever reason, they were in danger of homelessness, starvation and the workhouse, all misfortunes that could instigate madness.

George Alexander Nicholls was admitted to the Hanwell Asylum in 1860. This 43-year-old, Anglican, educated, single man considered sober and industrious, had been a clerk to a coal merchant and then a ship owner. He must have been very successful in his first job, or, more probably inherited some money. Coal merchants were an important trade at this time as coal was necessary for powering the steam railways, ships and industrial engines as well as for cooking and heating. In becoming a ship owner, George would have been an active trader. Victorian Britain was the world's most powerful trading nation in the world, doing business with Europe, India, Asia and America and competition between the many ship owners was fierce. Four years before his attack of insanity, he experienced 'financial difficulty', had his ships seized and sold which caused him to become very distressed and he began to read the Bible a great deal. At first, he read in his ordinary voice and then in a 'loud, theatrical, pompous manner, applying portions of the text, especially the psalms, to himself'. In 1858 he wrote to the Queen about his own and his family's affairs, attributing their problems to a conspiracy. Subsequently he wrote to the Bishop of London on ecclesiastical matters and frequently to ministers of the crown on political subjects. Christmas 1859, George was told that a picture of Christ 'looked like him' and he decided that he was Christ. He then wrote further letters to the Queen and other members of the Royal Family signing himself 'Jesus Christ'. His delusions of grandeur increased and he wrote love letters to the Princess Mary of Cambridge (1833–1897), cousin of Queen Victoria. Some letters he signed in his own name, others in the name of Christ. He was 'remonstrated with' for sending letters to the palace and he promised to desist. He kept his promise; however, he took every opportunity of meeting the royal carriages and attracting notice. Eventually, the police intervened and he was brought before the magistrate, who sent him to the workhouse, from there he went to Hanwell. As previously noted, general paralysis caused the symptoms exhibited by George. In his notes there is the suggestion that his could have been a case of congenital syphilis as it was recorded that he had an insane brother who was in Bethlem.

It must be stressed that religion and religious matters permeated all levels of Victorian life in a manner that is almost unimaginable today. Every form of schooling stressed the importance of religion and adherence to scripture. Children's stories, popular publications and the weekly sermon received in church made sure that the population was biblically literate, a fact that is clearly demonstrable in Victorian fiction. It was therefore a natural occurrence that a man or a woman who was suffering from mental health problems might interpret what was happening to them through the vocabulary of religion. Frequent references to possession by evil spirits and the power of the Devil were common in diabolical delusions, but there was a sharp contrast between the expressions of men and women, with men having more extreme and less introspective reactions to what they were experiencing. Men talked about the Devil covering them, or members of their family, in sulphur and imagined other vicious and aggressive scenes of diabolical retribution. Delusions about devils, witches and possession could lead to them being violent.

Masturbation as a cause of madness

Sometimes, underlying sexual reasons were blamed for a man's insanity. In March 1857, Thomas Probert, a single, 25-year-old attorney's clerk with a 'good education', was admitted to Bethlem hospital suffering from delusions. The reason given for instigating this attack of insanity was 'over attention to religious matters'. Probert was said to be unable to reason or reflect on a matter that had taken a firm hold on his mind. He believed that a spell had been cast on him by 'an old man possessed by demons'. When this old man pointed at Probert, he had fallen immediately under his power and had lost all sensation on the left side of his body. According to the certifying doctor, he could not be reasoned out of this delusion. Another doctor stated that Probert believed that his mind had been taken from him by a surgeon 'who had dealings with the Devil'. The mention of the surgeon's name greatly agitated him. A fuller report explained the background to his illness.

Apparently, the first symptoms of insanity showed themselves when Probert had nearly completed his articles with an attorney. He appeared to have lived a secluded life in a very small town where there was little or no society and to have latterly cultivated the acquaintance of an old man who was 'morbidly religious and weak-minded'. This man gained considerable influence over Probert and his delusions were associated with him. During a conversation on religious experiences, the old man pointed at Probert and told him that 'he had it in him'. This sentence appeared to have worked upon his mind until he conceived the impression that there was a mystical meaning in it. He still spoke of the influence it produced, depriving him of the use of the left side of his body. He was now in good health and industrious, but his strange beliefs still persisted. He confessed to having masturbated when younger, but not recently. After nearly three months in hospital, Probert's delusions were said to have faded and he was discharged, 'cured'.

The Victorian psychiatrist Henry Maudsley (1835–1918) believed that masturbating from an early age produced serious consequences to health, especially mental health. He described chronic masturbators as 'degenerate beings' whose physical and intellectual strength was damaged by this 'exhausting vice'. Other doctors, such as William Acton (1813–1875) and R.J. Brodie, who wrote *The Secret Companion: A Medical Work on Onanism* (1845), were vociferous in their condemnation of what was termed 'the solitary vice', as instigating masturbatory insanity. However, doctors also associated severe physical symptoms with masturbation and loss of sperm, believing it not only a cause of madness but also of blindness, epilepsy, sores, impotence, chronic fatigue and even premature death.

The Victorian man would have been conscious of the influences of religion pervading society. The church even had an impact on asylum life and was a powerful component of the inmates' lives.[23] Men would be taught that the 'spilling of seed' outside sexual intercourse between a married couple was a sin, and they would have been familiar with the story in Genesis 38, in which Onan was killed by God for spilling his seed when he withdrew from Tamar, his brother's widow, before he reached orgasm. As his seed was 'wasted', Onan became associated with masturbation and onanism was employed as a Victorian term for sexual self-abuse.[24] The idea that masturbation was forbidden by the Bible was confirmed by the words of surgeon Dr R.J. Brodie: 'We will endeavour to point out, on the sure and firm basis of scriptural authority, the evils, troubles, dissentions, heart-rendings and constitutional infirmities, resulting from impure and wanton pursuits.'[25]

In many male records, masturbation was indicated as a cause of insanity which could be cured by constant observation of the patient concerned, something that was made possible by the incarceration of the mad in county asylums. Because sexual arousal involved the stimulation of the nervous system, Victorian doctors concluded that masturbation might eventually undermine the health of the brain, diagnosing masturbation as a threat to sanity.

Brodie gives a 'medical' explanation of the danger of masturbation:

The seminal fluid is the very essence of the vital principle; – the most
essential part of the blood; – it is, in fact, the embryo of the species; – hence
the frequent repetition of the vice (masturbation) produces a wanton waste
and overflow of this most nutritious secretion, and brings on all the evils.[26]

A man's sperm was seen as a vital force and expressing it continually depleted
his energy. As Brodie put it:

Self-pollution is a habit so baneful to many, apparently approaching to years
of maturity, but who, alas! By their perverted inclinations, create a worm in
the core, which destroys the germ of manhood, and proves more destructive
than any disease to which the rising generation is liable; it entails the greatest
misery, and generates languor, debility, disease and weakness of mind,
instead of that vigour so essential to the purposes of life.[27]

He also stressed the way in which religion condemned the practice of self-
abuse, associating it with feelings of guilt and impiety. He stated:

There is not a place, either in the Old or New Testament, where uncleanliness,
the lust of the flesh or the abomination of Sodom are not condemned, but
this sin (masturbation) is hinted at amongst others and there is no doubt
but those who are guilty of it are comprehended among the abominable.
Who shall have their part in "lake which burneth with fire and brimstone."
– Rev.21,8.[28]

Often medics mixed their religious beliefs with their medical opinions.
Christians believed that human bodies were the temples of the Holy Spirit and
Brodie endorsed this belief saying that, therefore, 'we are bound to preserve
them in purity, and to employ them to holy purposes'.[29] It was because of this
link to religious teaching that Nathaniel Penrose, a sixteen-year-old, Primitive
Methodist teacher and preacher, was diagnosed in 1862 by the doctors at Colney
Hatch as suffering from 'religious excitement and addiction to masturbation'.
He was violent and believed that the Lord had given him faith but he had 'killed
many people', including his father. Nathaniel was described as being 'pallid
and feeble', having 'the look of one addicted to self-pollution' which he had
practised for some time. He had also been 'meddling dangerously in religion',
attempting to teach people before he had been properly taught himself.

The over-study of religion was often given as the underlying cause of men's madness. William Henry Sutcliff, a 24-year-old Quaker clerk, was admitted to Bethlem in October 1824 because he was suicidal. He refused to give any reason for his strange conduct and answered the questions put to him with just an occasional yes or no. He repeated 'short scriptural sentences', which had no relevance or connection to what was being said to him. He had 'a fixed, vacant look' and spent all his time, except meal times, in his room, mostly in the dark. Founded by George Fox (1624–1691), The Society of Friends, or Quakers, as they were known, had become more prominent in the nineteenth century, mainly due to their support of causes such as the abolition of slavery and prison reform. It was not easy to become a member of the Quakers in Victorian times; their silent worship and close-knit communities made them different from other Protestant groups. They did, however, consider the Bible a great inspirational book their beliefs instilled them with a social conscience. In 1796, William Tuke founded the York Retreat, a mental hospital that followed Quaker philosophy and refuted the, sometimes cruel, treatment of patients in other mental asylums.

Before his admittance, Sutcliff had refused to go out for air with anybody, as he believed that this would be a pleasure and therefore wrong. He did, however, keep trying to escape from his friends and family. Once he packed up all his belongings and put them in a cab with the intention of going somewhere quiet. On being stopped, he said he did not know where he was going, but watched for an opportunity and escaped over the garden wall and was away for several hours. His friends said that they were afraid that he had 'suicidal intentions' and that he was 'religiously incoherent'. The doctor in Bethlem observed that Sutcliff had been an intelligent clerk until the last few weeks when the symptoms of insanity showed themselves. He had been devoting all his spare time to the study of religion and this was reckoned to be the cause of his illness. The doctor concluded that although he had not been detected in the act, there was very little doubt that masturbation was the real cause. Sutcliff was discharged from Bethlem, cured, soon afterwards. Because the asylum records were not comprehensive, it was difficult to understand why the doctor came to the conclusion that William Sutcliff was suicidal because of his habit of masturbation rather than because of the influence of the Quaker religion. Whether he was 'caught in the act' or confessed was unknown. More likely, a sense of guilt consumed him, self-reproach generated by religious doctrine that held that masturbation was a sin and so psychological and consequences were inevitable. A term such as 'filthy habits' which was used by doctors to explain the reason for some Bethlem patients' violent behaviour would have only reinforced men's feelings of mortification.

Pretentious ideas linked to religion could be seen in men admitted to lunatic asylums diagnosed as suffering from religious excitement due to monomania on religion. Monomania had its origins in the work of the French psychiatrist Jean-Etienne Esquirol (1770–1840). In the nineteenth century it was a diagnosis of partial insanity in a patient who showed a single pathological preoccupation. Joseph Phillips Connell, a butcher aged eighteen, from Fish Street in the City of London was brought into Bethlem in May 1857 in a 'straight waistcoat', diagnosed with monomania but masturbation was also noted as a possible cause of his condition He was described as 'quite unmanageable'. He would not eat and was very agitated. Joseph believed himself to be 'chosen to preach the Gospel' and that 'the Lord would call him by a trumpet to minister to the Queen'. He gave his money away and neglected his business. He was treated with morphia, castor oil and an enema. This calmed him, but soon afterwards he became maniacal again. Whilst in this state, he was observed in the act of masturbation, which his doctors saw as a vital clue to his madness. The medical staff noted that his friends could 'assign no reason for his illness', but it turned out that he had been in the habit of masturbating for years. When maniacal, he was constantly practising self-abuse, and when he was rational he acknowledged the habit. Joseph Connell's behaviour was erratic, but he 'worked well in the hospital garden'. By July he was discharged, 'quite well'.

In Victorian England, two-thirds of all women and men with mental illness were classified as suffering from some sort of mania, the most loosely defined psychiatric classification because it covered so many conditions. Symptoms included extreme excitement, delusions, irrational behaviour and disordered thought.[30] The mid–late nineteenth century saw the sub-division of the more general term, mania, into the categories of senile, religious, puerperal and hysterical and noted the intensity by adjectives such as acute or partial. Men were not seen to suffer from hysterical mania and of course could not experience the puerperal kind. Both genders were diagnosed as experiencing religious mania but it manifested itself differently in men from how it appeared in women and it was extremely rare to find a hospital record that attributed the cause of mania in a woman to masturbation even when she might be suspected of indulging in the practice. More often, masturbating women were seen to be suffering from hysteria or nymphomania.

Emotion and religion

The link between the religious, emotional and sexual sides of man's nature was made by George Savage, superintendent of Bethlem Royal Hospital, in his book, *Insanity and Allied Neuroses: A Practical and Clinical Manual* (1884). He observed:

> We have to bear in mind that fact that religion is very closely allied to love, and that the love of woman and the worship of God are constant sources of trouble to unstable youth … the religious and sexual sides of man's nature are both closely connected with the emotional development and are both closely connected also with its organic nature. I have often been astonished to find that miserable patients in a lunatic asylum were still indulging in some form of sexual excess.[31]

This connection was illustrated by the case of Walter Cheesman, a timber merchant who was admitted to Bethlem Hospital being a 'danger to others'. The condition of this 27-year-old man was said to have been 'excited by both disappointed affection and religious delusions', caused by a broken engagement. Imagining that various individuals were 'incarnations of the Devil', he was under the illusion that he was being 'pursued by an army who had orders to take his life'. He was sometimes violent, had to be placed under restraint and had attempted to jump from the window at, what his keepers thought to be, an 'unreasonable time of night'. One of Walter's symptoms was that he liked to run away from home and hide himself in an orchard, though what he did there was not recorded. He continued to see devils under his bed and with whom he liked to converse. He affirmed that 'his medical attendant had died', passed through 'the torments of hell', and was returned. Consequently, he esteemed and respected this man. He was a stout, muscular man who sometimes, 'impulsively jumped from his seat where he had been sitting for some hours and broke a pane of glass or struck a fellow patient'. He talked generally with great energy and attempted to describe the torments of hell, of which he said 'he has had the opportunity of judging'. Cheesman was discharged from Bethlem 'uncured'. Whatever initially caused his madness and made him delusional and violent could, at this time, be expressed by the patient in terms of unrequited love and diabolical possession. This language was accessible to a Victorian timber merchant of 'moderate education' who was trying to make sense of the intensity of his mood swings and his outbreaks of actual physical violence. Walter's diabolical, religious delusions were very different from those experienced by female patients because of their violence and self-importance. Although he was suicidal, he did not blame himself for his situation.

Doctors recognized the links between violent, hysterical behaviour, religious fervour and sexual frustration. Henry Maudsley talked of what appeared to be deep religious feeling, arising from an unsatisfied sexual instinct. He said, 'The fanatic religious sects, which every now and then appear in in a community and disgust it by the offensive way in which they commingle religion and love, are really inspired by an uncontrolled and disordered sexual instinct.'[32] Maudsley was not talking about recognized Protestant groups here but of more extreme sects and false messiahs[33]; nevertheless, he clearly recognized how complex and powerful emotions could be exploited and even cause madness. He added, 'Without doubt, a hot religious perversion, and the earnest display of a feverish religious zeal, are, in some instances, really a phase in the manifestations of a morbid disposition, not unlikely to pass at some time into actual mental derangement.'[34]

It was not only the young who experienced sudden mental breakdowns, older men too became violent with religious delusions. George Hacon was forty-nine when he succumbed and became dangerous to himself and others. He was admitted to the asylum because of his 'great despondency, especially on religious subjects', his inclination to 'do someone mischief' and his using blasphemous language, something that was common in such cases. Having been previously a very active man he began to leave his work as an iron moulder to lie in bed for two to three days, then, unexpectedly, he would leave home and wander aimlessly around and threaten his wife. He believed himself to be completely mad and attempted suicide by drowning. Hacon was recorded as belonging to the Primitive Brethren which was a conservative, evangelical Christian movement that believed that Christianity should return to the practices and beliefs of the early apostolic church and take its teachings directly from biblical texts. His indoctrination by this movement may have affected his mental health. He 'worked well in the asylum garden', his depression lifted and he was discharged 'cured'. There was no further reference to his religious delusions following the judgement that these were what had 'excited' his condition. This case would concur with Leonard Smith's conclusion concerning the patients who filled nineteenth-century mental asylums when he stated that:

> The complex relationship between religion and insanity influenced many admissions. Religious zeal was socially acceptable to a point, but when construed as excessive the descent into madness was feared, manifested in gross over-activity or deluded ideas. References to figures like the Devil, the Holy Ghost or the Virgin Mary were common.[35]

As previously noted, the over-study of religion was believed to produce symptoms of madness and violence. The case of twenty-year-old Weslyan John Beck, a single house painter from Andover, demonstrated this conviction. Beck was a man of sober habits with a good education; the instigating cause of his condition was recorded as being 'over-study, especially religion'. Weslyanism is another name for Methodism as the movement was started by John Wesley (1703–1791). During the nineteenth century, itinerant preachers were renowned for their fiery, bordering on fanatical, sermons, which were considered dangerous to those with weak or over-receptive minds and could cause madness. Beck became increasingly aggressive and swore at and threatened any one whose beliefs differed from his. He easily lost control, quitting his employment because his master gave him 'a slight reproof'. He had 'exalted views' about himself and his personal piety which made him consign anybody who disagreed with him to 'eternal damnation'. The doctor in Bethlem described Beck as a respectable looking young man with no outward appearance of insanity. His disease was marked by an exaggerated idea that he was able to explain religious matters and texts in the Bible better than other people, something that was most likely the result of his following the teachings of the Methodist preachers who based their sermons on biblical texts and believed their understanding of the words of the New and Old Testaments superior to their fellow Christians. However, he accounted for this power by pronouncing he was supernaturally endowed. Beck was deemed cured of his obsession and discharged from the asylum.

Men suffering from religious mania or excitement manifested their psychological distress in a different way from women diagnosed with the same mental illness, noticeable in the language they used to express their difficult and inexplicable emotions. Men harnessed their religious beliefs in a manner that enabled them feel more important than they really were; their visions were often of self-aggrandisement and so frequently led to violence. Women, on the other hand, had a fear of hell and retribution that they were convinced they had brought about themselves through their sin. Because of their religious education, they blamed themselves for their visions and suffering. On scrutinizing the male admittance records during the middle years of the nineteenth century, a pattern of typical reasons for those admissions appeared. As noted, there was a certain masculinity attached to the instigating causes as men were admitted suffering from loss or stress of job, business going badly, over-study, excitement on the subject of the war with Russia (quite common in 1855), bankruptcy, gout, violent exercise and even excessive work and the effect of beer under a hot sun. When sex was the problem, their madness was usually due to onanism or masturbation. In contrast, the reasons for women's admissions were put down to emotional causes or failures in the female reproductive system. They were most likely to be driven mad by disappointment in love, seduction, having an illegitimate child, childbirth, menopause or uterine irritation.

Epilogue

But I was like a gentle lamb
Led to the slaughter.

Jeremiah 11.19

Religion and the services of the hospital chaplain formed a very important part of everyday life in a Victorian lunatic asylum, and the spiritual well-being of the inmates was deemed to be important in their treatment. Far from being seen as a possible origin of many delusions or the cause of women's sense of unworthiness, worship was perceived to be a comfort to the patients who were encouraged to attend services. A collection of sermons in two volumes with the title *Cheerful Words*, edited by William Hyslop, the proprietor of Stretton House Private Lunatic Asylum, was published in 1874 and was destined for the inmates of public institutions such as mental hospitals, workhouses and prisons. In his preface, Hyslop set out his purpose and supported his reasoning with a quote from Thomas Harrington Tuke (1826–1888), a British psychiatrist who ran the Manor House Asylum in Chiswick and specialized in non-restraint treatment:

> For many years I felt it to be my duty to prepare brief and simple discourses, which could be listened to and appreciated by patients suffering from varied types of mental disease. I have found such services very beneficial, and I am borne out in my conviction of their utility by one of the most distinguished of contemporary psychologists, Harrington Tuke, Esq., F.R.C.P., the President of the Medico-Psychological Association. In a brilliant address delivered before the association in August last, Mr. Tuke makes the following pertinent observations: – 'Close bonds knit together the duties of the Divine and the general physician; but in no branch of medicine, when admissible to all, is religious consolation more necessary than in the treatment of *mental depression* or *morbid fear;* no functions can be more closely united than those which require us firmly, yet trustfully, to attempt to heal those that are broken in heart, to give medicine to heal their sickness.'[1]

Tuke was an advocate for religious consolation, something that is still being discussed in mental health forums today.[2] Religion is often seen as supportive and beneficial to mental patients, but it has also been demonstrated that those who believe in a punishing God are more liable to experience poorer health outcomes than those who believe in a kind and non-judgemental one. This idea takes on a different cultural dimension when applied to nineteenth-century women, working-class women in particular. They were not made mad by religion, nor did they find much consolation from sermons such as those found in *Cheerful Words*. It would seem, from the records, that many females were deemed insane due to multiple and various causes and their distress led them to the conclusion that they were being punished by God. Even when they were experiencing physical pain, grief or hormonal changes brought about by childbirth, doctors frequently diagnosed them as suffering from religious delusions, mania or melancholy. If we look closely at girl's religious education, how they were taught that sin led to misery, their conviction that they were reaping punishment from God is explicable.

Guilt, lack of assertiveness and power, and their place in a patriarchal society made women in asylums vulnerable to invasive treatment and sexual abuse. Their voices frequently went unheard and unheeded by their relatives and the mind doctors. When they attempted to vocalize their mental or physical anguish, they used imagery they were most conversant with and because of this were diagnosed as suffering from religious excitement, mania, delusions, or monomania or some form of hysteria. Even though some female Victorian authors understood more about the causes of women's mental breakdowns, nineteenth-century literature was prone to demonize the unfeminine madwoman and infantalize the more innocent, simpleminded 'girl'. Men in lunatic asylums reflected Victorian ideas on masculinity and femininity, especially the male doctors' analyses and opinions on mental health. These medical judgements were important in the way that madwomen and madmen were assessed and treated.

Beliefs expressed by Victorian mind doctors were not mere curiosities from bygone days, but fundamentally they represented the unspoken content of much modern psychiatry.[3] Nineteenth-century doctors demonstrated an attitude that would most likely be repudiated by psychiatrists today but which, in actuality, represents much of their approach to therapy. What has changed over the years is the way in which women are treated for their diagnosed mental illnesses. Today they are subdued by psychotropic drugs, given counselling and other therapies and sometimes incarcerated in specialist psychiatric hospitals or units of mainstream hospitals when they are considered to be of danger to themselves or others. The way in which women express their mental distress has also changed; in recent years, their anxieties are more likely to reflect the fears and beliefs of the twenty-first century rather than those of the nineteenth century. However, beneath the vocabulary and historically related expressions of suffering, the unhappiness, rebellion and physical pain would appear to remain the same as it ever was. Madness has its own vernacular, depending on the century in which it is being written or spoken about and it is important to decipher the meaning behind the idiom and how it differed when used by men and women. Today, we have a very different approach to understanding the suffering of the mentally ill and this can cloud our perception of what the nineteenth-century patient was experiencing

The Victorian alienist, W. Browne (1805–1885), summed up the association between madness and religion in his lectures delivered before the managers of the Montrose Lunatic Asylum:

Wherever lunatics are collected together, a great many cases are always designated religious, and supposed to be attributable to enthusiasm. This partly proceeds from the difficulty of obtaining correct information as to the history of each case, and partly from the philosophical blunder of concluding that in insanity the cause is invariably of the same nature as the effect. ...

I am convinced from observation, that although this *cause* does not operate more powerfully, the number of religious maniacs is greater in Britain than elsewhere. The explanation is obvious. Religion has here its due exercise and awful importance; the mind is trained, thinks and feels under its influence; and when from misfortune or ambition, or physical injury, the place of reason is usurped, it may always be predicated, first that the delusions which succeed will correspond to the natural disposition, and secondly to those impressions which have been most powerful and permanent; and hence there are not a greater number of maniacs; but there are a greater number of maniacs exhibiting a certain class of delusions, because our countrymen are, whatever may be their errors, naturally and habitually devout.[4]

Because they were 'habitually devout' and biblically literate, the language employed by females to describe their psychological and spiritual torments led the mad doctors to consider that they were experiencing religious 'excitement' and delusions. To suffer the depths of melancholia or to undergo the horrors of mania or suicidal thoughts and ideation must have left these unfortunate women sincerely believing that they were indeed lost souls.

Notes

Preface

1   Charlotte Brontë, *Jane Eyre* (Oxford: Oxford University Press 2000) 12.
2   Ibid., p. 15.
3   For example, see: Colin Gale and Robert J Howard, *Presumed Curable: An Illustrated Casebook of Victorian Psychiatric Patients in Bethlem Hospital* (Petersfield: Wrighton Biomedical Publishers Ltd. 2003).
4   Roy Porter, *Madness* (Oxford: Oxford University Press 2002) 158.
5   Darian Leader, *What Is Madness?* (London: Penguin Books 2012) 7.
6   Barbara Taylor, *The Last Asylum* (London: Penguin Books 2015) Prologue.

Chapter 1

1   A large proportion of private asylums were located in the London area, and they mainly catered for small numbers of inmates.
2   For a more comprehensive history of Bethlem Hospital, see Patricia Allderidge, *Bethlem Hospital 1247–1997: A Pictorial Record* (Chichester, West Sussex: Phillimore & Co. Ltd 1997). Catherine Arnold, *Bedlam: London and Its Mad* (London: Simon & Schuster 2008). Andrew Scull, Charlotte MacKenzie and Nicholas Hervey, *Masters of Bedlam: The Transformation of the Mad-Doctoring Trade* (Princeton, NJ: Princeton University Press 1996).
3   Elaine Showalter, 'Victorian Women and Insanity', in *Victorian Studies* vol. 23 Winter (Bloomington, IN: Indiana University Press 1980).
4   Robert Brudnell Carter, *On the Pathology and Treatment of Hysteria* (London: John Churchill 1853) 25.
5   Ibid., p. 26.
6   Ibid., p. 67.
7   Dr John Conolly (1794–1866) was a pioneering psychiatrist at the Middlesex County Asylum at Hanwell, from 1839. He was one of the first mind doctors to

regard an asylum as a hospital which had patients who were treated, rather than inmates who were restrained.

8   Elaine Showalter, *The Female Malady: Women, Madness and Culture, 1830–1980* (London: Virago Press 1987) 79.

9   Re-printed in, Jeffrey Moussaieff Masson, *A Dark Science: Women, Sexuality and Psychiatry in the Nineteenth Century* (New York: Farrar, Strauss & Giroux 1986) 44–59.

10   Wiliam Niederland, *The Schreber Case* (New York: Quadrangle Books 1974) and 'Schreber and Flechsig: A Further Contribution to the "Kernel of Truth" in Schreber's Delusional System', *Journal of American Psychoanalytic Association* 16 (1968): 740–8.

11   A magazine edited by Charles Dickens, published 1850–1859.

12   Charles Dickens, *Household Words*, January 1852.

13   William Willis Mosely, 'Predisposing and Exciting Causes of Insanity'. (Excerpt from, *Eleven Chapters on Nervous and Mental Complaints*) (London: Simpkin, Marshall & Co., 1838) 123–40. Cited in Vieda Skulkans, *Madness and Morals: Ideas on Insanity in the Nineteenth Century* (London: Routledge & Keegan Paul 1975) 49.

14   See, George H. Savage, *Insanity and Allied Neuroses* (London: Cassel, 1884) 53.

15   The study is found in Chapter 4 of this book.

16   John Conolly M.D. D.C.L., *The Character of Insanity*. A Lecture Delivered before the Royal Institution of Great Britain. May 1854.

17   'A Constant Observer', in *Sketches in Bedlam: or Characteristic Traits of Insanity* (London: Sherwood Jones & Co., 1823) 278–9.

18   Michel Foucault, *Madness and Civilisation: A History of Insanity in the Age of Reason*, trans. Richard Howard (London: Routledge, 1997) 255–7.

19   Quoted in: Denis Leigh (Physician, The Bethlem Royal and Maudsley Hospitals London) *The Historical Development of British Psychiatry. Vol 1 18th. and 19th. Centuries* (London: Pergamon Press Ltd. 1961) 233.

20   Marit Fimland, 'On the Margins of the Acceptable: Charlotte Brontë's *Villette*', *Literature & Theology* 10, no. 2 (June 1996): 148–59. Fimland argues that in *Villette*, Lucy Snowe narrates her own story of solitude, companionship, love and loss, and she tries to make sense of her own experience and her own life. In doing so, she refers to typologically different biblical texts, and she relates them to her own life. In this way she emphasizes and interprets different aspects of her own existence. She sees this as Brontë writing with the Bible in her bones.

Chapter 2

1   Henry Maudsley, *The Physiology and Pathology of Mind* (London: Macmillan and Co. 1868) 274.

2   Ibid., p. 341.

3   John Haslam, *Considerations on the Moral Management of Insane Persons* (London: R. Hunter 1817) 4–5.

4   For further explanation see: Diana Peschier, *Nineteenth-Century Anti-Catholic Discourses: The Case of Charlotte Brontë* (Hampshire: Palgrave Macmillan 2005). Chapter 3.

5   Quotation by ex-Roman Catholic priest Blanco White, printed on the cover of *The Indelicacy of Auricular Confession as Practised by the Roman Catholic Church: Correspondence between Hon. George Spencer and Rev. E. Riland Bedford* (Birmingham: William Hodgetts, 1836).

6   Charles Darwin, *The Descent of Man* (New York: D. Appleton 1875) 557.

7   Londa Schiebinger, 'Skeletons in the Closet: The First Illustrations of the Female Skeleton in Eighteenth-Century Anatomy', *Representations*, no. 14 Spring (University of California Press 1986).

8   Alfred Beaumont Maddock, *The Education of Women*. Excerpt from *Practical Observations on Mental and Nervous Disorders* (London: Simpkin and Marshall & Co. 1854) 16–17.

9   See, Sylvia M Barnard, *To Prove I'm Not Forgot: Living and Dying in a Victorian City* (Stroud, Gloucestershire: The History Press 2009) Chapter 4, in which Maddock is described as a thoughtful and amiable man.

10 Elaine Showalter, *The Female Malady*, p. 79.

11 See Chapter 1, p. 4. The ideas of Dr John Conolly 1794–1866.

12 Leonard D Smith, *Cure Comfort and Safe Custody: Public Lunatic Asylums in Early Nineteenth-Century England* (London: Leicester University Press 1999) Chapter 3, Waste Stuff: Peopling the Asylum.

13 Colin Gale and Robert T Howard, *Presumed Curable: An Illustrated Casebook of Victorian Psychiatric Patients in Bethlem Hospital* (Petersfield Hampshire: Wrightstone Biomedical Publishing Ltd. 2003). Louise Hide, *Gender and Class in English Asylums, 1890–1914* (Basingstoke: Palgrave Macmillan 2014). Kathryn Burtinshaw and John RF Burt, *Lunatics, Imbeciles and Idiots: A History of Insanity in Nineteenth-Century Britain and Ireland* (Barnsley: Pen and Sword Books 2017).

14 Judith Walzer Leavitt, ed., *Women and Health in America* (Wisconsin: University of Wisconsin Press 1999) Diagnosing Unnatural Motherhood: Nineteen-Century Physicians and 'Puerperal Insanity' Nancy Theriot.

15 See Hilary Marland, *Dangerous Motherhood: Insanity and Childbirth in Victorian Britain* (Basingstoke: Palgrave Macmillan 2004).

16 George H. Savage, *Insanity and Allied Neuroses Practical and Clinical* (London: Cassell and Co. 1884) 24–5.

17 Ibid., p. 377.

18 For a more comprehensive explanation and statistics, see: I. Loudon, 'Puerperal Insanity in the Nineteenth Century', *Journal of The Royal Society of Medicine* 81 (February 1988): 76–9.

19 David Berguer, *The Friern Hospital Story: The History of a Victorian Lunatic Asylum* (London: Chaville Press 2012).

20 Infant mortality was high during the nineteenth century. It averaged about150 deaths per 1,000 live births. This statistic was often higher in areas of rapid urbanization, such as London.

21 See Dorothy L. Haller's Paper: *Bastardy and Baby Farming in Victorian England* (New Orleans: Loyola University 1989).

22 Charles Dickens, *Oliver Twist,* Chapter 1. 1839.

23 Prior to 1834, unmarried mothers had been legally entitled to support from the fathers of their children. After 1834, they could only receive help by going into the workhouse. The new law was supposed to act as a deterrent to bastardy, as a woman would be less inclined to engage in pre-marital sex if she knew she would be held solely responsible for any resultant children. However, the Bastardy Clause did not have the desired effect and there was an increase in cases of infanticide and abandonment.

24 Since the 1990s, 'Battered Woman/Wife Syndrome' has been a recognized psychological state. Women with this syndrome believe that they deserve the abuse they receive and cannot escape from it. During the nineteenth century this would not have been recognized because of the Victorian, misogynistic culture.

25 Taken from: *Eleven Chapters on Nervous and Mental Complaints* (London: Simpkin, Marshall & Co. 1838) 123–40.

26 George H. Savage, *Insanity and Allied Neuroses: A Practical and Clinical Manual* (London: Cassell and Co. Ltd. 1884) 56–7.

27 See Jennifer Wallis' article, 'This Fascinating and Fatal Illness', in *The Psychologist, the Journal of the British Psychological Society*, October 2012.

28 'A Constant Observer'.

29 Jane Ussher, *Women's Madness: Misogyny or Mental Illness?* (Amherst Massachusetts: University of Massachusetts Press 1991) 3.

30 See, Louise L Jackson, *Child Sexual Abuse in Victorian England* (London: Routledge 2000) 25.

31 Because of privacy rules concerning mental health records that are held in the Republic of Ireland today, the names of the women concerned have to remain secret.

32 John Mitford, *A Description of the Crimes and Horrors in the Interior of Warburton's Private Madhouse, Commonly Called Whitmore House* (London: Benbow 1825) 2.

33 Ibid., p. 3.

34 Ibid., p. 17.

35 See: Diana Peschier *Nineteenth Century Anti-Catholic Discourses.* Chapters 2 and 3.

36 John Mitford, *A Description of the Crimes and Horrors in the Interior of Warburton's Private Madhouse at Hoxton.*

37 'The Alleged Lunatics' Friend Society was founded in 1838, becoming an official society in 1845. It was an advocacy group started by former asylum patients, including glass manufacturer Lewis Phillips who had been in Warburton's house, and their supporters. The society campaigned for greater protection against wrongful confinement, cruel and improper treatment and for the reform of the lunacy laws.

38 John Mitford, *A Description of the Crimes and Horrors in the Interior of Warburton's Private Madhouse at Hoxton*, p. 15.

39 Ibid., p. 16.

40 *Jeremiah* 11.19.

Chapter 3

1 Charles Williams L.R.C.P. L.R.C.S L.S.A. *Religion and Insanity* (London: The Ambrose Co. 1909).

2 Dr George H. Savage, *Insanity and Allied Neuroses: Practical and Clinical* (London: Cassell 1884) 50–1.

3 See Chapter 4 for a more detailed explanation.

4 The twenty-first-century American psychologist Gail Hornstein recognized the need to listen to first-person narratives written by people who were deemed

mad. She detected a code present in the writing of the mentally ill and attempted to explain their 'madness' from within. Gail A Hornstein, *Agnes's Jacket: A Psychologist's Search for the Meaning of Madness* (Herefordshire: PCCS Books 2012).

5   Michel Foucault, *Madness and Civilisation*, pp. 255–7.

6   Letter from Mr James Bigg found by the author tucked into the Female Case Notes for Hanwell Hospital 1858.

7   Sir W.C. Ellis M.D., *A Treatise on the Nature, Symptoms, Causes and Treatment of Insanity with Practical Observations on County Lunatic Asylums and a Description of Pauper Lunatic Asylums for the County of Middlesex at Hanwell, with a Detailed Account of Its Management* (London: Samuel Holdsworth 1838) 67.

8   Ibid.

9   Ibid.

10 Ibid.

11 A.L. Wiggins M.D., *A New View of Insanity. The Duality of the Mind Proved by the Structure, Functions and Diseases of the Brain and by the Phenomena of Mental Derangement and Shewn to Be Essential to Moral Responsibility* (London: Longman, Brown, Green and Longmans 1844) 427.

12 Ibid.

13 Ibid., p. 432.

14 George H. Savage M.D. F.R.C.P. *Insanity and Allied Neuroses: A Practical and Clinical Manual* (London: Cassell & Co. 1884) 32.

15 See, Charlotte Brontë, Letter to Ellen Nussey Brussels, 2 September 1843, reproduced in, Juliet Barker, *The Brontës: A Life in Letters* (London: Viking 1997) 116.

16 Also see the case of Ellen Penfold in Chapter 2.

17 Henry Maudsley, *The Physiology and Pathology of Mind*, p. 384.

18 Lawrence Babb, *Sanity in Bedlam: A Study of Robert Burton's Anatomy of Melancholy* (Westport, CT: Greenwood Press 1977).

19 Images 8 & 9 (Fanny Smith).

20 For further explanation of the importance of historical context to delusion see: David Wright, 'Delusions of Gender? Lay Identification and Clinical Diagnosis of Insanity in Victorian England', in *Sex and Seclusion, Class and Society: Perspectives on Gender and Class in the History of British and Irish Psychiatry*, ed. Jonathan Andrews and Anne Digby (Amsterdam and New York: Rodopi 2004) 166–7.

21 Charlotte Brontë, *Villette* 1853, eds. Margaret Smith and Herbert Rosengarten (Oxford: Oxford University Press, 2000) 495.

22 Ibid., p. 495.

23 George Savage, the prominent nineteenth-century psychiatrist, expressed the opinion that religious excitement might produce some insanity by unhinging the minds of young, nervous females who had experienced the unsettling experience of a 'religious wave'.

Chapter 4

1 *The Child's Guide* was supposed to represent Carus Wilson's publication *The Children's Friend*.

2 In order to encourage regular attendance at Sunday school, children would be rewarded for reaching certain 'milestones' in their education. These rewards were often books with an uplifting and moral theme which could be borrowed by or given to a diligent pupil.

3 Elizabeth Gaskell, *The Life of Charlotte Brontë 1857* (London: Penguin Books 1985) 107.

4 H. Shepheard, *A Vindication of the Clergy Daughter's School and of the Rev. Carus Wilson* (Kirby Lonsdale: Robert Morphet and London: Seeley, Jackson & Halliday 1857).

5 The Brontës lived in the parsonage in Haworth, a village in West Yorkshire. Their father Patrick was the local rector.

6 M.J. Quinlan, *The Victorian Prelude: A History of English Manners 1700-1830* (New York: Columbia University Press 1941) 112–13. Cited in P.B. Cliff, *The Rise and Development of the Sunday School Movement in England 1780–1980* (Redhill: National Christian Education Council 1986) 78.

7 Ibid., p. 76.

8 T.W. Laqueur, *Religion and Respectability: Sunday Schools and Working Class Culture 1780–1850* (London: Yale University Press 1976) 142.

9 *The Teacher's Visitor* was a journal for Sunday School teachers containing advice on what to teach and how to instil evangelical, morality into their pupils. It was edited by Rev. W.C. Wilson.

10 Ibid., p. 142.

11 For a literary viewpoint, see Mrs Gaskell's novel *Ruth* (1853) in which the dissenting author points out the hypocrisy of the doctrine of original sin when it is used against an innocent, illegitimate child born of a misused, young mother.

12 Charlotte Brontë, *Jane Eyre 1847* (Oxford: Oxford University Press 2000) 32.

13 Ibid., pp. 63–7.

14 George Eliot, 'The Evangelical Teaching of Dr. Cumming', *Westminster Review*, October 1855.

15 For a comprehensive view of the debate, see F.M.L. Thompson, 'Social Control in Victorian Britain', *The Economic History Review* 2nd Series 34, No. 2 (May 1981): 189–208.

16 Quinlan, *Victorian Prelude*, p. 41 and pp. 44–50. Cited in Laqueur, *Religion and Respectability*, p. 182.

17 E.P Thompson, *The Making of the English Working Class* (London: Pelican Books 1968) 9–11.

18 T.W. Laqueur, *Religion and Respectability*.

19 Ibid.

20 Thomas H. Gallaudet, *The Child's Book of the Soul* (London: Seeley and Sons 1832).

21 Ibid.

22 Clara Lucas Balfour, *Women Worth Emulating*, Sunday School Presentation Book (Frome, Somerset and London: Butler & Tanner, The Selwood Printing Works 1817) preface.

23 Verse attributed to 'Dodderidge', cited in A Female Teacher, *Hints to Girls on Dress: Especially Intended for Scholars in Daily and Sunday Schools* (London: Religious Tract Society 1836).

24 Ibid.

25 Ibid., p. 20.

26 *A Lily among the Thorns, or, Short Memorials of Little Jane* (London: Wertheim & Macintosh 1856).

27 A Female Teacher, *Hints to Girls on Dress*, p. 12.

28 *Mary Meanwell and Kitty Pertly, or, The Effects of Vanity. A Tale Written for the Use of Girls in Sunday School* (Bath: S. Hazard 1799) 38.

29 Matilda Planche, *The Children's Sunday Album*, or *Short Stories for Sunday Reading* (London: Cassell, Petter and Galpin 1848).

30 *The Child's Companion*, or *Sunday Scholar's Reward* (London: Religious Tract Society 1824).

31 The act of stealing apples.

32 *The Happy Life. A Gift for Sunday Schoolgirls* (London: Jarrold and Sons 1850) 12–13.

33 Ibid., p. 22.

34 The Rev. W. Carus Wilson, *The Children's Friend* (Kirby Lonsdale: Carus Wilson 1845).

35 Written by Albert Midlane 1859.

36 In *Religion and Respectability,* Laqueur suggests that many writings on this subject were formulaic.

37 Rev. W. Carus Wilson, *Youthful Memoirs of a Little Girl Who Died in Oxfordshire* (Philadelphia: American Sunday School Union 1829).

38 Elizabeth Gaskell, *North and South* (London: Everyman, J.M. Dent 1993) 136. Chapter 17.

39 Michael Wheeler, *Death and Future Life in Victorian Literature and Theology* (Cambridge: Cambridge University Press 1990) 25.

40 *Jane Eyre,* Chapter. 9.

41 Memoir of Sarah Becker 11 years old, *The Children's Friend*, December 1826, p. 78.

42 Matilda Planche, *The Children's Sunday Album.*

43 Jane Ewbank, *The Life of William Carus Wilson 1791–1859* (Kendal: Titus Wilson & Son 1960) 24.

44 Anon, *The Young Servant's Friendly Instructor*, Religious Tract Society (London: R. Clay Printer 1835) 21.

45 Ibid.

46 Ibid.

47 Michael Wheeler, *Death and the Future Life in Victorian Literature and Theology,* (Cambridge: Cambridge University Press 1990) 182–5.

Chapter 5

1 Poem reproduced in Edwin Fuller Torrey and Judy Miller, *The Invisible Plague: The Rise of Mental Illness from 1750 to the Present* (London: Rutgers University Press 2002).

2 Jane Ussher, *The Psychology of the Female Body* (London: Routledge 1989) 3.

3 Edward Jukes, *Indigestion and Costiveness with Hints to Both Sexes* (London: Simpkin and Marshall 1831) 27–8.

4 William Hewett, *On Costiveness: Its Causes, Consequences and Cure* (London: George Philip and Son 1865) 35.

5 For example, Isaac Baker Brown's case no. 1 (1859) page 15 of this chapter.

6 George H. Savage, *Insanity and Allied Neuroses*, pp. 84–5.

7 The notion of hysteria resulting in catalepsy was somewhat sent up by Charles Dickens in *Bleak House* (1852–1853) when Mrs Snagsby, convinced that her husband has been hiding the fact that the crossing keeper Jo is his illegitimate

son, works herself into an hysterical state of spasms and shrieking that leads to the onset of catalepsy. She becomes so rigid that she has to be carried upstairs like a grand piano (*Bleak House* chapter 25).

8   Robert Brudnell Carter, 1828–1918, was an English physician and ophthalmic surgeon who wrote *On the Pathology and Treatment of Hysteria*, 1853.

9   Brudnell Carter, *On the Pathology and Treatment of Hysteria*, pp. 2–3.

10 For a fuller explanation of monomania see, Stewart, Lindsey 2018 *Monomania: The Life and Death of a Psychiatric Idea in Nineteenth-Century Fiction 1836–1860*. PhD Thesis, The Open University.

11 As Bethlem had no means of restoring Mary to health, even though she had been fed and rested, she would have fallen into the category 'uncured' and made to leave the hospital.

12 Researchers at the Co. Cork archives are forbidden from using the names of the inmates of mental hospitals even when the records are over 100 years old.

13 It had to be presumed that the hospital mentioned here was the hospital wing of the asylum as there was no mention of her being discharged to another institution.

14 As in the case of Martha Higgins in Chapter 5.

15 George H. Savage M.D. *Insanity and Allied Neuroses: Practical and Clinical*. Chapter iv, p. 46.

16 An 'exciting cause' meant something that initiated the attack of madness.

17 Savage, *Insanity and Allied Neuroses*. Ch. iv, p. 46.

18 Dr John Charles Bucknill 1817–1897 was an English psychiatrist and mental health reformer. He founded *The Asylum Journal* in 1853, which became *The Journal of Medical Science* in 1858.

19 Dr John Charles Bucknill, 'Modes of Death Prevalent among Insane', *America Journal of Insanity* 19, no. 3 (January 1863): 354–62. (First published in *The Journal of Mental Science* ed. John Charles Bucknill).

20 Today, the close relationship between skin disease and mental health is well documented. The All Party Parliamentary Group on Skin titled, *The Psychological and Social Impact of Skin Diseases on People's Lives* 2013 set out the detrimental effects a skin disorder could have on the mental health of the sufferer.

21 Diaper was the Victorian word for sanitary towel/rags.

22 For further explanation of religious fasting girls and women in history, see: Rudolph M. Bell, *Holy Anorexia* (London & Chicago: The University of Chicago Press 1987).

23 Henry Maudsley, *The Physiology and Pathology of Mind*, p. 515.

24 See Lisa Appignanesi, *Mad, Bad and Sad: A History of Women and the Mind Doctors from 1800 to the Present* (London: Virago 2009) 435–8.

25 'Young women searching for an idiom in which to say things about themselves focused on food and the body. Some middle class girls, then as now, became preoccupied with expressing an idea of female perfection and moral superiority through denial of appetite.' J. Brumberg, *Fasting Girls: The Emergence of Anorexia Nervosa as a Modern Disease* (Cambridge, MA: Harvard University Press 1988) 188.

26 Smith, W. Tyler, 'The Climacteric Disease in *Women*', *London Journal of Medicine* 1 (1848): 601 Quoted in Elaine Showalter, *The Female Malady*, p.75.

27 Ibid.

28 See Alexander Morison, *Outlines on Lectures on the Nature, Causes and Treatment of Insanity* (London: Longmans, Brown, Green & Longmans 1848).

29 Brudnell Carter, *On the Pathology and Treatment of Hysteria*, pp. 25–6.

30 Ibid., p. 33.

31 William Acton, *The Functions and Disorders of the Reproductive Organs, in Childhood, Youth, Adult Age and Advanced Life, Considered in Their Physiological, Social and Moral Relations* (London: Churchill 1862).

32 Isaac Baker Brown, *On the Curability of Certain Forms of Insanity, Epilepsy, Catalepsy, and Hysteria in Females* (London: Robert Hardwicke 1866) 3.

33 Ibid., p. 4.

34 Ibid., p. 4.

35 Dr Henry Monro, 'On the Nomenclature of the Various Forms of Insanity', *Asylum Journal Mental Science* 2, no. 17 (1856): 286–305.

36 See: Jean Stengers and Anne Van Necck, *Masturbation: The History of a Great Terror* (New York: St. Martin's Press 2001); and Tom Laqueur, *Solitary Sex: A Cultural History of Masturbation* (Cambridge, MA: Zone Books 2004).

37 The letter was discovered by the author. It was tucked in to the Colney Hatch female case book for 1859 next to the record of patient number 2113, Sarah Rebecca Thorley.

38 See, Leonore Davidoff, *Worlds Between: Historical Perspectives on Gender & Class* (Cambridge: Polity Press 1995) 109.

39 John Millar, *The Dangers of Masturbation*, in *Hints on Insanity* (London: Henry Renshaw 1861) 37–40.

40 See, www.lesleyahall.net, 'Victorian Sex Factoids', *Clioridectomy*.

41 Ibid.

42 A euphemism for masturbation.

43 Baker Brown, *On the Curability of Certain Forms of Insanity*, p. 8.

44 Elaine Showalter, *The Female Malady*, pp. 72–3.

45 Hannah Claridge, Colney Hatch 1870, was diagnosed as suffering from mania following a serious operation for breast cancer. She died a painful death in a mental asylum.

Chapter 6

1 John Conolly, *On Some Forms of Insanity* (London: Savill and Edwards 1849).

2 Mrs Gaskell, *The Poor Clare* in *The Manchester Marriage and Other Stories 1851* (Stroud, Gloucestershire: Alan Sutton Publishing Ltd. 1990) 163.

3 Elizabeth Gaskell, *Cousin Phillis* (London: Penguin Books 2004) 304.

4 Ibid., p. 308.

5 Ibid., p. 309.

6 Thomas Hardy, *Tess of the D'Ubervilles* 1891 Chapter 14. (Hertfordshire: Wordsworth Editions 1993) 82.

7 A quotation attributed to 11 Peter 2:3 *Tess of the D'Urbervilles* chapter 12, p. 70.

8 Ibid., pp. 70–1.

9 Ibid., p. 71.

10 Elaine Showalter, *The Female Malady*, p. 61.

11 Mr Robert Gardiner Hill 1811–1878, surgeon.

12 Rosina Bulwer Lytton, *A Blighted Life: A True Story* (London: Swan, Sonnenschein, Lowrey & Co. 1887) 4.

13 Ibid., p. 5.

14 John Mitford, *A Description of the Crimes and Horrors in the Interior of Warburton's Private Madhouse* at Hoxton, p. 30.

15 Brontë, *Jane Eyre*, p. 305.

16 Ibid.

17 Ibid.

18 Andrew Wynter, *The Borderlands of Insanity: And Other Allied Papers* (London: Robert Hardwicke 1875) 52.

19 Mary Elizabeth Braddon, *Lady Audley's Secret* 1861–1862 (Oxford: Oxford University Press 1992) 346.

20 Ibid., p. 348.

21 Ibid., p. 349.

22 Ibid., p. 350.

23 Ibid., p. 350.

24 Mrs Henry Wood, *St. Martin's Eve: A Novel* (London: Richard Bentley & Son 1885).

25 Exodus 34: 6–7.

26 Brontë, *Villette*, p. 273.

27 *Jane Eyre,* Volume ii Chapter ii, p. 177.

28 In 1838, the psychiatrist Alexander Morison published a book, *The Physiognomy of Mental Diseases*. It contained plates of psychiatric patients with brief case descriptions. In the same year, the French psychiatrist, Esquirol, also used psychiatric illustrations in his book, *Of Mental Diseases*. See, Sander L. Gilman, ed., *The Face of Madness: Hugh Diamond and the Origin of Psychiatric Photography* (Brattleboro, VT: Echo Books 2014) Introduction.

29 Jane Eyre, Volume ii Chapter ii, p. 177.

30 Henry Maudsley, *The Physiology and Pathology of Mind*, p. 478.

31 Ibid., p. 479.

32 George H. Savage, *Insanity and Allied General Neuroses* (Philadelphia: Henry C Lea's Son & Co. 1884) 152–3.

33 Ibid., p. 152.

34 See, Leonore Davidoff, *Worlds Betweeen: Historical Perspectives on Gender and Class* (Oxford: Polity Press 1995) 109.

35 Kathryn Hughes, *The Victorian Governess* (London: The Hambleton Press 1993) 1.

36 Barker, *The Brontës*, p. 65.

37 Ibid., p. 66.

38 For a fuller explanation of how governesses were perceived in the nineteenth century see Kathryn Hughes, *The Victorian Governess*.

39 See Henry Maudsley, *Body and Mind* (London: Macmillan & Co. 1873) 79–80.

40 See George Man Burrows, *Commentaries on Insanity* (London: Underwood 1828) 191–3.

41 See Charcot, J.M., 'Sur les localizations cérébrales', *Comptes-Rendus des Seánces et Mémoires de la Société de Biologie* 24 (1875): 400–4. Charcot, J.M. *Lectures on the Diseases of the Nervous System, Delivered at La Salpêtrière* (London: New Sydenham Society 1877). Charcot, J.M., 'Physiologie pathologique. Sur les divers états nerveux déterminés par l'hypnotisation chez les hystériques. [Pathological Physiology: On the Various Nervous States Determined by the Hypnotisation of Hystericals]', *Comptes rendus de l'Académie Des Sciences* 94 (1882): 403–5. Charcot, J.M., *Oeuvres complètes.* [Complete works] (Paris: Bureau du Progrès Mèdical 1885).

42 Flaubert took his definition of hysteria from his father's copy of the *Dictionnaires des Sciences Médicales* (1824). In *Madame Bovary*, Dr Bovary has this book on the bookshelf in his surgery.

43 Wilkie Collins, *Jezebel's Daughter* (Stroud: Alan Sutton Publishing 1995) 19.

44 Mesmerism was a method of psychological healing developed by the Viennese doctor Franz Anton Mesmer 1734–1815. It was originally known as animal magnetism. Mesmerism produced a trance-like state in the patient, but was different from hypnotism being non-verbal. It remained popular until the end of the nineteenth-century and because of the influence the practitioner exerted over the recipient, it was the cause of some unease.

45 John Sutherland, *Victorian Fiction: Writers, Publishers, Readers* (Basingstoke: Macmillan 1995) 77–80.

46 Taken from *The Journal of Pathological Medicine and Mental Pathology* October 1860, p. 457.

47 See the case of Caroline Brent, Chapter 5, p. 11.

48 See The case of Elizabeth James, Chapter 2, p. 14.

49 Conolly, *On Some Forms of Insanity*.

50 *Jane Eyre*, volume 1 Chapter X11, p. 109.

51 *Jane Eyre*, volume 11 Chapter V111, p. 253.

52 *Lady Audley's Secret*, Chapter V11, pp. 52–3.

53 Rev. John Jessop, *Woman* (London: A.M. Pigott 1851) 27.

54 Mary Elizabeth Braddon, *Lady Audley's Secret*, p. 387.

55 Ibid., p. 392.

56 Charles Dickens, 'The Lazy Tour of Two Idle Apprentices Chapter the Fourth'. *Household Words* 24 October 1857. Re-printed in: *Charles Dickens: 'Gone Astray' and Other Papers from Household Words 1851–59*, ed. Michael Slater (London: J.M. Dent 1998).

57 Ibid., pp. 448–9.

Chapter 7

1 Edward Henry Bickersteth, *Yesterday, Today and Forever* 1866. Epic poem on Hades, Paradise and Hell. Quoted in Michael Wheeler, *Death & the Future Life in Victorian Literature and Theology* (Cambridge: Cambridge University Press 1990) 176.

2 See, Michael Roper and John Tosh, eds., *Manful Assertions: Masculinities in Britain since 1800* (London: Routledge 1991) 2.

3 Andrew Scull, ed., *W.F. Browne and the Mid-Nineteenth-Century Consolidation of Psychiatry* (London: Tavistock/Routledge 1991) 67.

4 Ibid.

5 These men were portrayed in literature as characters like Sidney Kirkwood in George Gissing's *The Nether World* (1889), who was kind, diligent and behaved in a Christian manner.

6 Arthur Morrison, *A Child of the Jago*, in *Tales of The Old London Slums* (E-artnow 2016) chapter 7.

7 J.G. Millingen, *Aphorisms on Insanity* (London: John Churchill 1840) 8.

8 See Janet Oppenheim, *Shattered Nerves: Doctors, Patients, and Depression in Victorian England* (Oxford: Oxford University Press 1996) 141–58.

9 The proprietor of Whitmore House Asylum in Hoxton where Mitford spent some time.

10 John Mitford, *A Description of the Crimes and Horrors of Warburton's Private Madhouse at Hoxton*, pp. 10–14.

11 Henry 'Orator' Hunt (1773–1835) was a British radical speaker who advocated parliamentary reform and the repeal of the Corn Laws. He was one of the speakers at the rally in Manchester in 1819 which turned into the 'Peterloo Massacre'. He was subsequently arrested and spent two years in prison.

12 John Mitford, *A Description of the Crimes and Horrors of Warburton's Private Madhouse at Hoxton*, pp. 10–14.

13 See Elizabeth Stephens, 'Spermatorrhoea, the Lesser Known Version of Hysteria', in *The Conversation* (online journal) (2012).

14 George Savage, *Insanity and Allied Neuroses*, p. 46.

15 For the Victorian doctor's ideas on constipation, or costiveness, and how it affected mental health, see Chapter 1, p. 1.

16 Henry Maudsley, *The Physiology and Pathology of Mind*, pp. 262–3.

17 Andrew Wynter, *The Borderlands of Insanity*, p. 266.

18 Ibid., p. 69.

19 Ibid., p. 70.

20 George Savage, *Insanity and Allied Neuroses*, p. 337.

21 In his article 'Delusions of Gender?', David Wright admitted that men were more prone to delusions of grandeur than women. See David Wright, 'Delusions of Gender?'

22 See Leonore Davidoff and Catherine Hall, *Family Fortunes: Men and Women of the English Middle Class 1780–1850* (London: Routledge 1992) 230.

23 See C.T. Andrews, *The Dark Awakening: A History of St. Lawrence's Hospital Bodmin* (London: Cox & Wyman 1978) 138.

24   See Julie Peakman, *The Pleasure's All Mine: A History of Perverse Sex* (London: Reaktion Books 2013) chapter 2.

25   Dr R.J. Brodie, *The Secret Companion: A Medical Work on Onanism* (London: Brodie R.J. & Co., Consulting Surgeons 1845) vi.

26   Ibid., p. 11.

27   R.J. Brodie, *The Secret Companion,* p. 10.

28   Ibid., p. 12.

29   Ibid., p. 13.

30   David Wright, 'Delusions of Gender?' p. 164.

31   George H. Savage M.D. F.R.C.P. Late physician and superintendent of Bethlem Royal Hospital, *Insanity and Allied Neuroses: A Practical and Clinical Manual* (London: Cassell and Co. 1884) 55–6.

32   Henry Maudsley, *The Physiology and Pathology of Mind,* p. 240.

33   Such as spiritualism or the sect of the Agapemonites, founded by Henry Price in 1846.

34   Ibid., p. 241.

35   Leonard D. Smith, *Cure, Comfort and Safe Custody: Public Lunatic Asylums in Early Nineteenth Century England* (London: Leicester University Press. 1999) 102.

Epilogue

1   Ed. William Hyslop, proprietor of Stretton House Private Lunatic Asylum for gentlemen. Shropshire Church Stretton, *Cheerful Words: Sermons, Specially Adapted for Delivery Before Inmates of Lunatic Asylums, Unions, Workhouses, Hospitals, Gaols, Penitentiaries, and Other Public Institutions* (London: Messrs. Bailliere, Tindall and Cox 1874) Preface.

2   See Kate M. Loewenthal and Christopher Alan Lewis, 'Mental Health, Religion and Culture', *The Psychologist, Journal of the British Psychological Society* 24 (April 2011): 256–9.

3   See Mossaieff Masson, *A Dark Science.*

4   'What Asylums were, are and ought to be': being the substance of five by W.A.F. Browne surgeon, medical superintendent of the Montrose Lunatic Asylum, formerly president of the Royal Medical Society, Edinburgh. In Andrew Scull, ed., *The Asylum as Utopia: W.F. Browne and the Mid-Nineteenth Century Consolidation of Psychiatry* (London: Tavistock/Routledge 1991) 34–5.

Bibliography and Sources

Primary Sources

Female Casebooks:

Bethlem Royal Hospital 1850–60. Bethlem Museum of the Mind: CB- 049-077 series box no. A04/7 series CB.

1870–3: CB- 097-103 series box no. A01/5 series CB.

Broadmoor Criminal Lunatic Asylum 1864–5. Berkshire County Records Office: D/H/14/D

City of London Mental Asylum 1866–7. London Metropolitan Archives: CLA/001/B/01/001

Colney Hatch Lunatic Asylum (2nd Middlesex County Asylum) 1850–60, 1870–74, 1893–5. London Metropolitan Archives: H12/CH/B/11/1-42.

Cork Mental Hospital, District Lunatic Asylum (Our Lady's Hospital) Ireland 1870–80. Cork City and Archives Service: OLH/65 boxes 8,9,11,12.

1894–1900: OLH/66 boxes 1–4.

Essex County Lunatic Asylum 1880–1890. Essex County Records Office: A/H 10/2/5/1-6.

Fair Mile Hospital, Berkshire County Lunatic Asylum 1871–74. Berkshire County Records Office: DH/10/D/2

Hanwell Pauper and Lunatic Asylum (1st Middlesex County Asylum) 1830–70. London Metropolitan Archives: H11/HLL/B/19/001-019.

Ticehurst House Mental Hospital, Sussex 1860–65. Wellcome Library: mss 6361-6499.

Male Casebooks:

Bethlem Royal Hospital 1857–59. Bethlem Museum of the Mind: CB-070 series box no. AO/3/4 series CB.

Hanwell Pauper and Lunatic Asylum 1854–77. London Metropolitan Archives: H11/Hll/B/20/003/4-13.

Colney Hatch Lunatic Asylum (2nd Middlesex County Asylum) 1855–62. London Metropolitan Archives: H12/CH/B/13/ 5–6.

William Acton, *The Functions and Disorders of the Reproductive Organs, in Childhood, Youth, Adult Age and Advanced Life, Considered in Their Physiological Social and Moral Relations* (London: Churchill 1862).

Anon, *Mary Meanwell and Kitty Pertly, or, the Effects of Vanity: A Tale Written for the Use of Girls in Sunday School* (Bath: S. Hazard 1799).

Anon, *The Happy Life: A Gift for Sunday Schoolgirls* (London: Jarrold and Sons 1850).

Anon, *A Lily among the Thorns, or, Short Memorials of Little Jane* (London: Wertheim & Macintosh 1856).

Matthew Arnold, *The Buried Life* 1852.

Isaac Baker Brown, *On the Curability of Certain Forms of Insanity, Epilepsy, Catalepsy and Hysteria in Females* (London: Robert Hardwicke 1866).

Clara Lucas Balfour, *Women Worth Emulating*. Sunday School Presentation Book (London: 1817).

Edward Henry Bickersteth, *Yesterday, Today and Forever*. Epic Poem on Hades, Paradise and Hell 1866.

Mary Elizabeth Braddon, *Lady Audley's Secret* 1861–2 (Oxford: Oxford University Press 1992).

Dr. R.J. Brodie, *The Secret Companion: A Medical Work on Onanism* (London: Brodie R.J. & Co. Consulting Surgeons 1845).

Charlotte Brontë, *Letter to Ellen Nussey*, Brussels 2 September 1843.

Charlotte Brontë, *Jane Eyre* 1847 (Oxford: Oxford University Press 2000).

Charlotte Brontë, *Villette* 1853 (Oxford: Oxford University Press 2000).

Robert Brudnell Carter, *On the Pathology and Treatment of Hysteria* (London: Churchill 1853).

Rosina Bulwer-Lytton, *A Blighted Life* (London 1880).

Robert Burton, *The Anatomy of Melancholy* 1621.

William Hyslop (ed.), proprietor of Stretton House Private Lunatic Asylum for Gentlemen. Church Stretton, Shropshire, *Cheerful Words: Sermons, Specially Adapted for the Delivery before Inmates of Lunatic Asylums, Unions, Workhouses, Hospitals, Gaols Penitentiaries and Other Public Institutions* (London: Messrs. Bailliere, Tindall and Cox 1874).

The Child's Companion, or Sunday Scholar's Reward (London: Religious Tract Society 1824).

Wilkie Collins, *The Woman in White* 1860 (London: Penguin Classics 2003).

Wilkie Collins, *Jezebel's Daughter* 1880 (Stroud: Alan Sutton Publishing 1995).

John Conolly, *On Some Forms of Insanity* (London: Savill and Edwards 1849).

John Conolly, *The Character of Insanity*. A Lecture Delivered before the Royal Institution of Great Britain (May 1854).

'A Constant Observer', *Sketches in Bedlam: or Characteristic Traits of Insanity* (London: Sherwood Jones & Co. 1823).

Caleb Crowther, *Observations on the Management of Madhouses* (London: Simpkin, Marshall and Co. 1841).

Charles Dickens, *Oliver Twist*, 1839 (Oxford: Oxford University Press 1966).

Charles Dickens, *Household Words*, January 1852.

Charles Dickens, *Bleak House*, 1852–3 (London: Penguin Books 1985).

Charles Dickens, *The Lazy Tour of Two Idle Apprentices. Chapter the Fourth* in *Household Words*, 24 October 1857.

Emily Dickinson, *One Need Not Be a Chamber to Be Haunted*, 1862.

Dr. Direx, *Women's Complete Guide to Health* (New York: Townsend and Adams 1869).

George Eliot, 'The Evangelical Teaching of Dr. Cumming', *The Westminster Review*, October 1855.

Sir W.C. Ellis, *A Treatise on the Nature, Symptoms, Causes and Treatment of Insanity with Practical Observations on County Lunatic Asylums and a Description of Pauper Lunatic Asylums for the County of Middlesex at Hanwell, with a Detailed Account of Its Management* (London: Samuel Holdsworth 1838).

A Female Teacher, *Hints to Girls on Dress: Especially Intended for Scholars in Daily and Sunday Schools* (London: Religious Tract Society 1836).

Gustav Flaubert, *Madame Bovary* 1856 (Oxford: Oxford University Press 2008).

Elizabeth Gaskell, *Ruth* 1853 (London: Penguin Books 1997).

Elizabeth Gaskell, *North and South* 1855 (London: Penguin Books 1996).

Elizabeth Gaskell, *The Life of Charlotte Brontë* 1857 (London: Penguin Books 1985).

Elizabeth Gaskell, *The Poor Clare* 1859 (Stroud Gloucestershire: Alan Sutton Publishing Ltd. 1990).

Elizabeth Gaskell, *Cousin Phillis* 1864 (London: Penguin Books 2004).

Thomas H. Gallaudet, *The Child's Book of the Soul* (London: Seeley and Sons 1832).

George Gissing, *The Nether World* 1889 (Oxford: Oxford University Press 2008).

Thomas Hardy, *Tess of the D'Urbervilles* 1891 (Hertfordshire: Wordsworth Editions 1993).

John Haslam, *Considerations on the Moral Management of Insane Persons* (London: R. Hunter 1817).

William Hewitt, *On Costiveness: Its Causes, Consequences and Cure* (London: George Philip and Son 1865).

William Hyslop (ed.), *Cheerful Words: Sermons, Specially Adapted for Delivery before Inmates of Lunatic Asylums, Unions, Workhouses, Hospitals, Gaols, Penitentiaries and Other Public Institutions* (London: Messrs. Bailliere, Tindall and Cox 1874).

Rev. John Jessop, *Woman* (London: A.M. Piggott 1851).

Edward Jukes, *Indigestion and Costiveness with Hints to Both Sexes* (London: Simpkin and Marshall 1831).

Stewart Lindsey 2018 *Monomania: The Life and Death of a Psychiatric Idea in Nineteenth-Century Fiction 1836–1860*. PhD Thesis the Open University.

Alfred Beaumont Maddock, *The Education of Women* in *Practical Observations on Mental and Nervous Disorders* (London: Simpkin and Marshall & Co. 1854).

Henry Maudsley, *The Physiology and Pathology of Mind* (London: Macmillan & Co. 1868).

John Millar, 'The Dangers of Masturbation' in *Hints on Insanity* (London: Henry Renshaw 1861).

J.G. Millingen, *Aphorisms on Insanity* (London: John Churchill 1840).

John Mitford, *A Description of the Crimes and Horrors in the Interior of Warburton's Private Madhouse at Hoxton, Commonly Called Whitmore House* (London: Benbow 1825).

Sir Alexander Morison, *Outlines on Lectures on the Nature, Causes and Treatment of Insanity* (London: Longmans, Brown, Green and Longmans 1848).

Arthur Morrison, *A Child of the Jago* 1896 in *Tales of The Old London Slum* (E-artnow 2016).

William Willis Moseley, 'Predisposing and Exciting Causes of Insanity' Excerpt from, *Eleven Chapters on Nervous and Mental Complaints* (London: Simpkin, Marshall & Co. 1838).

Matilda Planche, *The Children's Sunday Album, or, Short Stories for Sunday Reading* (London: Cassell, Petter and Galpin 1848).

George H. Savage, *Insanity and Allied Neuroses: A Practical and Clinical Manual* (London: Cassell and Co. 1884).

H. Shepheard, *A Vindication of the Clergy Daughter's School and of the Rev. Carus Wilson* (Kirby Lonsdale 1857).

Michael Slater (ed.), *Charles Dickens: 'Gone Astray' and Other Papers from Household Words 1851–59* (London: J.M. Dent 1998).

A.L. Wiggins, *A New View of Insanity. The Duality of the Mind Proved by the Structure, Functions and Diseases of the Brain and by the Phenomena of Mental Derangement and Shewn to Be Essential to Moral Responsibility* (London: Longman, Brown Green and Longmans 1844).

Charles Williams, *Religion and Insanity* (London: The Ambrose Co. 1909).

Rev. W. Carus Wilson, *Youthful Memoirs of a Little Girl Who Died in Oxfordshire* (Philadelphia: American Sunday School Union 1829).

Rev. W. Carus Wilson, *The Children's Friend* (Kirby Lonsdale: 1826 and 1845).

Mrs. Henry Wood, *St. Martin's Eve: A Novel* (London: Richard Bentley & Son 1885).

Andrew Wynter, *The Borderlands of Insanity* (London: Robert Hardwicke 1875).

Anon, *The Young Servant's Friendly Instructor*, Religious Tract Society (London: R. Clay Printers 1835).

Secondary Sources

Patricia Allderidge, *Bethlem Hospital 1247–1997 A Pictorial Record* (Chichester, West Sussex: Phillimore & Co. Ltd. 1997).

C.T. Andrews, *The Dark Awakening: A History of St. Lawrence's Hospital Bodmin* (London: Cox & Wyman 1978).

Jonathan Andrews and Ann Digby (eds.), *Sex and Seclusion, Class and Society: Perspectives on Gender and Class in the History of British and Irish Psychiatry* (Amsterdam and New York: Rodopi 2004).

Lisa Appignanesi, *Mad, Bad and Sad: A History of Women and the Mind Doctors from 1800 to the Present* (London: Virago 2009).

Catherine Arnold, *Bedlam: London and Its Mad* (London: Simon & Schuster 2008).

Lawrence Babb, *Sanity in Bedlam: A Study of Robert Burton's Anatomy and Melancholy* (Westport Connecticut: Greenwood Press 1977).

Juliet Barker, *The Brontës: A Life in Letters* (London: Viking 1997).

Sylvia M Barnard, *To Prove I'm Not Forgot: Living and Dying in a Victorian City* (Stroud, Gloucestershire: The History Press 2009).

Rudolf M. Bell, *Holy Anorexia* (London and Chicago: The University of Chicago Press 1987).

David Berguer, *The Friern Hospital Story: The History of a Victorian Lunatic Asylum* (London: Chaville Press 2012).

J. Brumberg, *Fasting Girls: The Emergence of Anorexia Nervosa as a Modern Disease* (Cambridge MA: Harvard University Press 1988).

Kathryn Burtinshaw and John R.F. Burt, *Lunatics, Imbeciles and Idiots: A History of Insanity in Nineteenth-Century Britain and Ireland* (Barnsley: Penn and Sword Books 2017).

Max Byrd, *Visits to Bedlam: Madness and Literature in the Eighteenth Century* (Columbia South Carolina: University of South Carolina Press 1975).

P.B. Cliff, *The Rise and Development of the Sunday School Movement in England 1790–1980* (Redhill: National Christian Education Council 1986).

Leonore Davidoff and Catherine Hall, *Family Fortunes: Men and Women of the English Middle Classes 1780–1850* (London: Routledge 1992).

Leonore Davidoff, *Worlds Between: Historical Perspectives on Gender and Class* (Cambridge: Polity Press 1995).

Jane Ewbank, *The Life of William Carus Wilson 1791–1859* (Kendal: Titus Wilson & Son 1960).

Marit Fimland, 'On the Margins of the Acceptable: Charlotte Brontë's *Villette*', *Literature and Theology*, vol. 10, June 1996.

Michel Foucault, *Madness and Civilisation: A History of Insanity in the Age of Reason*, trans. Richard Howard (London: Routledge 1997).

Colin Gale and Robert J. Howard, *Presumed Curable: An Illustrated Casebook of Victorian Psychiatric Patients in Bethlem Hospital* (Petersfield: Wrighton Biomedical Publishers Ltd. 2003).

Sander L. Gilman, *The Face of Madness: Hugh Diamond and the Origin of Psychiatric Photography* (Brattleboro, Vermont: Echo Books 2014).

Dorothy L. Haller, *Bastardy and Baby Farming in Victorian England* (New Orleans: Loyola University 1989).

Louise Hide, *Gender and Class in English Asylums, 1890–1914* (Basingstoke: Macmillan 2014).

Gail A. Hornstein, *Agnes's Jacket: A Psychologist's Search for the Meaning of Madness* (Hertfordshire: PCCS Books 2012).

Kathryn Hughes, *The Victorian Governess* (London: The Hambleton Press 1993).

Louise L. Jackson, *Child Sexual Abuse in Victorian England* (London: Routledge 2000).

T.W. Laqueur, *Religion and Respectability: Sunday Schools and Working Class Culture 1780–1850* (London: Yale University Press 1976).

T.W. Laqueur, *Solitary Sex: A Cultural History of Masturbation* (Cambridge Massachusetts: Zone Books 2004).

Darian Leader, *The New Black: Mourning, Melancholy and Depression* (London: Penguin Books 2008).

Darian Leader, *What Is Madness?* (London: Penguin Books 2012).

Denis Leigh, *The Historical Development of British Psychiatry,* vol. 1 (London: Pergamon Press Ltd. 1961).

Kate M. Loewenthal and Christopher Alan Lewis, 'Mental Health, Religion and Culture', *The Psychologist, Journal of the British Psychological Society*, vol. 24 April 2011.

Norman Longmate, *The Workhouse: A Social History* (London: Pimlico 2003).

Steven Marcus, *The Other Victorians: A Study of Sexuality and Pornography in Mid-Nineteenth Century England* (London: Weidenfeld and Nicholson 1966).

Hilary Marland, *Dangerous Motherhood: Insanity and Childbirth on Victorian Britain* (Basingstoke Hampshire: Palgrave Macmillan 2004).

Jeffrey Moussaieff Masson, *A Dark Science: Women, Sexuality and Psychiatry in the Nineteenth Century* (New York: Farrar, Strauss and Giroux 1986).

Janet Oppenheim, *Shattered Nerves: Doctors Patients and Depression in Victorian England* (Oxford: Oxford University Press 1996).

Julie Peakman, *The Pleasure's All Mine: A History of Perverse Sex* (London: Reaktion Books 2013).

Diana Peschier, *Nineteenth-Century Anti-Catholic Discourses: The Case of Charlotte Brontë* (Basingstoke: Palgrave Macmillan 2005).

Roy Porter, *The Faber Book of Madness* (London: Faber and Faber 1991).

Roy Porter, *Madness* (Oxford: Oxford University Press 2002).

Yannick Ripa, *Women and Madness: The Incarceration of Women in Nineteenth-Century France*, trans. Catherine Du Peloux Menage (Cambridge: Polity Press 1990).

Michael Roper and John Tosh (eds.), *Manful Assertions: Masculinities on Britain since 1800* (London: Routledge 1991).

Londa Schiebinger, 'Skeletons in the Closet: The First Illustrations of the Female Skeleton in Eighteenth-Century Anatomy', *Representations* no.14 Spring (University of California Press 1986).

Andrew Scull, *Museums of Madness: The Social Organisation of Insanity in Nineteenth-Century England* (London: Penguin Books 1979).

Andrew Scull (ed.), *The Asylum as Utopia: W. F. Browne and the Mid-Nineteenth Century Consolidation of Psychiatry* (London: Tavistock/Routledge 1991).

Andrew Scull, Charlotte MacKenzie and Nicholas Hervey, *Masters of Bedlam: The Transformation of the Mind-Doctoring Trade* (Princeton, NJ: Princeton University Press 1996).

Elaine Showalter, 'Victorian Women and Insanity', *Victorian Studies* Vol. 23, Winter (Bloomington, NJ: Indiana University Press 1980).

Elaine Showalter, *The Female Malady: Women, Madness and English Culture, 1830–1980* (London: Virago Press Ltd. 1987).

Vieda Skulkans, *Madness and Morals: Ideas on Insanity in the Nineteenth Century* (London: Routledge & Keegan Paul 1975).

Leonard D. Smith, *Cure Comfort and Safe Custody, Public Lunatic Asylums in Early Nineteenth-Century England* (London: Leicester University Press 1999).

William Styron, *Darkness Invisible: A Memoir of Madness* (London: Vintage Books 2004).

John Sutherland, *Victorian Fiction, Writers, Publishers, Readers* (Basingstoke: Macmillan 1995).

Barbara Taylor, *The Last Asylum: A Memoir of Madness in our Times* (London: Penguin Books 2015).

Edwin Fuller Torrey and Judy Miller, *The Invisible Plague: The Rise of Mental Illness from 1750 to the Present Day* (London: Rutgers University Press 2002).

E.P. Thompson, *The Making of the English Working Class* (London: Pelican Books 1968).

F.M.L. Thompson, 'Social Control in Victorian Britain', *The Economic History Review* second series, vol. 34 no. 2 May 1981.

Jane Ussher, *The Psychology of the Female Body* (London: Routledge 1989).

Jane Ussher, *Women's Madness: Misogyny or Mental Illness?* (London: Harvester Wheatsheaf 1991).

Wendy Wallace, *The Painted Bridge* (London: Simon and Schuster 2012).

Jennifer Wallace, 'This Fascinating and Fatal Illness', *The Psychologist*, the Journal of the British Psychological Society 2012.

Judith Walzer Leavitt (ed.), *Women and Health in America* (Wisconsin: University of Wisconsin Press 1999) Diagnosing Unnatural Motherhood: Nineteenth-Century Physicians and 'Puerperal Insanity'. Nancy Theriot.

Michael Wheeler, *Death and Future Life in Victorian Literature and Theology* (Cambridge: Cambridge University Press 1990).

David Wright, *Mental Disability in Victorian England: The Earlswood Asylum 1847–1901* (Oxford: Clarendon Press 2011).

Index